CRANIOFACIAL STRUCTURES IN CONNECTIVE TISSUE DISORDERS

FOR MARCH OF DIMES BIRTH DEFECTS FOUNDATION

Birth Defects Compendium, Second Edition, Daniel Bergsma, *Editor*

BIRTH DEFECTS: ORIGINAL ARTICLE SERIES

1986 — Volume 22

No. 3 **Prospective Studies on Children With Sex Chromosome Aneuploidy,** Shirley G. Ratcliffe and Natalie W. Paul, *Editors*

1987 — Volume 23

No. 1 **Genetic Aspects of Developmental Pathology,** Enid F. Gilbert and John M. Opitz, *Editors*

No. 2 **Genetic Risk, Risk Perception, and Decision Making,** Gerry Evers-Kiebooms, Jean-Jacques Cassiman, Herman Van den Berghe, and Géry d'Ydewalle, *Editors*

No. 3 **Medical and Experimental Mammalian Genetics: A Perspective,** Victor A. McKusick, Thomas H. Roderick, Joe Mori, and Natalie W. Paul, *Editors*

No. 5A **Thalassemia: Pathophysiology and Management, Part A,** Suthat Fucharoen, Peter T. Rowley, and Natalie W. Paul, *Editors*

No. 5B **Thalassemia: Pathophysiology and Management, Part B,** Suthat Fucharoen, Peter T. Rowley, and Natalie W. Paul, *Editors*

1988 — Volume 24

No. 1 **Retinopathy of Prematurity: Problem and Challenge,** John T. Flynn and Dale L. Phelps, *Editors*

No. 2 **Recent Advances in Ectodermal Dysplasias,** Carlos F. Salinas, John M. Opitz, and Natalie W. Paul, *Editors*

No. 4 **Anorectal Malformations in Children: Update 1988,** F. Douglas Stephens and E. Durham Smith, *Editors*

March of Dimes Birth Defects Foundation
Birth Defects: Original Article Series, Volume 25, Number 4, 1989

CRANIOFACIAL STRUCTURES IN CONNECTIVE TISSUE DISORDERS

Proceedings of the Tenth Annual Symposium of the Society of Craniofacial Genetics: A Symposium in Recognition of Dr. David Bixler Held in Baltimore, July 10, 1988

Editors
Jaime L. Frias, MD
University of Nebraska
Omaha, Nebraska

Natalie W. Paul
March of Dimes
Birth Defects Foundation
White Plains, New York

Assistant Editor
Victoria Sears Leonardo, MPH
University of Nebraska
Omaha, Nebraska

WILEY-LISS, NEW YORK

To enhance medical communication in the birth defects field, the March of Dimes Birth Defects Foundation publishes the *Birth Defects Compendium* (2nd Edition), an *Original Article Series*, a *Reprint Series*, *Nursing Staff Development Modules*, *Genetics in Practice* (a quarterly newsletter), and provides a series of films and related brochures.

Further information can be obtained from:

Professional Services Department
March of Dimes Birth Defects Foundation
1275 Mamaroneck Avenue
White Plains, New York 10605

Published by:
Alan R. Liss, Inc.
41 East 11th Street
New York, New York 10003

Views expressed in articles published are the authors', and are not to be attributed to the March of Dimes Birth Defects Foundation or its editors unless expressly so stated.

Library of Congress Cataloging-in-Publication Data

Society of Craniofacial Genetics. Symposium (10th : 1988 : Baltimore, Md.)
Craniofacial structures in connective tissue disorders : proceedings of the Tenth Annual Symposium of the Society of Craniofacial Genetics : a symposium in recognition of Dr. David Bixler held in Baltimore, July 10, 1988 / editors, Jaime Frias, Natalie W. Paul.
p. cm.—(Birth defects, original article series ; v. 25, no. 4)
At head of title: March of Dimes Birth Defects Foundation.
Includes bibliographical references.
ISBN 0-471-56688-8
1. Connective tissue—Diseases—Complications and sequelae—Congresses. 2. Head—Abnormalities—Congresses. 3. Genetic disorders—Congresses. 4. Bixler, David—Congresses. I. Bixler, David. II. Frias, Jaime. III. Paul, Natalie W. IV. March of Dimes Birth Defects Foundation. V. Title. VI. Series: Birth defects original article series ; v. 25, no. 4.
[DNLM: 1. Connective Tissue Diseases—congresses. 2. Face—abnormalities—congresses. 3. Skull—abnormalities—congresses. W1 BI966 v. 25 no. 4 / WE 705 S678c 1988]
RG626.B63 vol. 25, no. 4
[RC924]
616′.043 s—dc20
[616.7′7]
DNLM/DLC
for Library of Congress 89-12159
CIP

The March of Dimes Birth Defects Foundation is dedicated to the goals of preventing birth defects and ameliorating their consequences for patients, families, and society.

As part of our efforts to achieve these goals, we sponsor, or participate in, a variety of scientific meetings where all questions relating to birth defects are freely discussed. Through our professional education program we speed the dissemination of information by publishing the proceedings of these and other meetings. From time to time, we also reprint pertinent journal articles to help achieve our goals. Now and then, in the course of these articles or discussions, individual viewpoints may be expressed that go beyond the purely scientific and into controversial matters. It should be noted, therefore, that personal viewpoints about such matters will not be censored but this does not constitute an endorsement of them by the **March of Dimes Birth Defects Foundation**.

Contents

Contributors

David Bixler, DDS, Department of Oral Facial Genetics, Indiana University School of Dentistry, Indianapolis, IN 46223 **[3]**

Michael M. Cohen, Jr., DMD, PhD, Department of Oral Pathology, Faculty of Dentistry, Dalhousie University, Halifax, Nova Scotia, Canada **[39]**

Jaime L. Frias, MD, Department of Pediatrics, University of Nebraska Medical Center, Omaha, NE 68105-1065 **[xi,83]**

Robert J. Gorlin, DDS, MS, Department of Oral Pathology & Genetics, University of Minnesota School of Dentistry, Minneapolis, MN 55455 **[39]**

Gary Greenberg, PhD, School of Dentistry, University of Southern California, Los Angeles, CA 90089-0641 **[15]**

Michael Melnick, DDS, PhD, Craniofacial Biology Department, School of Dentistry, University of Southern California, Los Angeles, CA 90089-0641 **[1,15]**

Cedric Minkin, PhD, School of Dentistry, University of Southern California, Los Angeles, CA 90089-0641 **[15]**

John M. Opitz, MD, Department of Medical Genetics, Shodair Children's Hospital, Helena, MT 59601 **[27]**

Andrew E. Poole, DDS, PhD, Department of Pediatric Dentistry and Craniofacial Disorders Team, University of Connecticut Health Center, Farmington, CT 06032 **[73]**

Robyn Rosenstein, DDS, School of Dentistry, University of Southern California, Los Angeles, CA 90089-0641; present address: 200 East Chestnut Street, Chicago, IL 60611 **[15]**

John J. Sauk, DDS, Department of Pathology, Dental School, University of Maryland, Baltimore, MD 21201 **[7]**

Ioan T. Thomas, MD, Department of Pediatrics, Bowman Gray School of Medicine, Winston-Salem, NC 27103 **[83]**

The numbers in brackets are the opening page numbers of the contributors articles.

Preface

In 1979 the Society of Craniofacial Genetics and the March of Dimes Birth Defects Foundation co-sponsored a symposium on the developmental aspects of craniofacial dysmorphology, to foster "much needed communication between clinical dysmorphologists and developmental biologists." This was the beginning of a tradition that has continued successfully through a decade. The articles compiled in this book attest to this fact. As program chairman, I am delighted to present to you the proceedings of the Tenth Symposium of the Craniofacial Genetics Society, which covered different clinical and basic aspects of the craniofacial structure in connective tissue disorders.

I wish to express my appreciation to the distinguished speakers, who made this conference an outstanding scientific event. It is also with gratitude that I recognize the support of the March of Dimes Birth Defects Foundation, the Bureau of Maternal and Child Health and Resources Development, and Ross Laboratories, whose support made possible the meeting and the publication of these proceedings. The secretarial assistance of Joan Rostermundt is acknowledged with praise.

The symposium was dedicated to David Bixler—eminent clinician, outstanding scientist, and superior human being—in recognition of his enormous contributions to the Society and to the study of craniofacial anomalies.

Jaime L. Frias, MD

In Honor of David Bixler

Michael Melnick, DDS, PhD

Craniofacial Biology Department, School of Dentistry, University of Southern California, Los Angeles, CA 90089-0641

In anxious and uncertain times like ours, when it is difficult to find pleasure in humanity and the course of human affairs, it is a particularly pleasurable task to say a few personal words about such a superior and quiet man as David Bixler. Indeed it is an honor.

In this enterprise we call biomedical science, there are many schools of thought that govern our approach to human development, many and varied persons within each school, and, perhaps, just as many motives that have led each of us to our own special thematic commitments. Were some czar to come along with the sole purpose of driving out all of us who entered the scientific enterprise for intellectual sport as a way to satisfy egotistical ambition or material reward, few would be left to engage the important questions. One of these few would be David Bixler, and that is why we who know him well love him. Unlike most of us, David could not have been anything other than what he is, a scientist, a man with a mission, a man with integrity.

To have been a student of David's was a privilege and a stroke of good fortune, for he is the model teacher. Whatever I have achieved myself as a professor I owe in largest measure to David's tutelage. David Bixler got it right. He never told us what to do, instead he taught us how to do it. He gave us the tools to make empiric observation in our naive quest for some new knowledge. But his insight and great value as a mentor goes far beyond that. He taught us how to uncover a measure of truth from the observations we had recorded.

Unlike most teachers he first taught us that thoroughness brought great reward even if it temporarily put one at a disadvantage relative to those in the fast lane of grant-getting and publishing. But beyond this, he taught us that scientific truth was not dogma. Although a cautious and conservative man by nature, David taught us to reject the notion of truth as correspondence. With David, one was not forced to make the observed data fit the current wisdom. Rather, David taught us that truth in science must always be contingent with the facts regardless of what the majority believes. David has spent countless

Birth Defects: Original Article Series, Volume 25, Number 4, pages 1–2

hours with all of us who studied with him, prodding us to be certain that what we concluded to be the truth was indeed contingent with our observations.

David Bixler's accomplishments in craniofacial genetics and dysmorphology are numerous and of great quality. Most of you here know them and I need not recount them today. Suffice it to say that David Bixler is one of the founding fathers of craniofacial genetics and has maintained continuous NIH funding for more than two decades, a remarkable record indeed. His former students populate the core of the workers in this field, and many of them are here today.

For all of us, to honor David with this excellent symposium today is but a small measure of our gratitude to him for all he has done for us. For David Bixler, it is a most fitting beginning to another decade of important research and wise counsel. If anyone of us has half the impact on this field that David has had, we will certainly judge ourselves successful.

David, we thank you for putting up with us over the years and wish you all the best in the future. We *need* you!

Acknowledgment and Comments

David Bixler, DDS, PhD

Department of Oral Facial Genetics, Indiana University School of Dentistry, Indianapolis, IN 46223

I would like to acknowledge gratefully the recognition that the Society of Craniofacial Genetics and its officers has bestowed on me and my work at this time.

On this occasion, which is also the tenth anniversary of the annual meeting of the Society of Craniofacial Genetics, and because the Society officers have assembled such a highly qualified panel of speakers to present craniofacial research topics at this meeting, I take the opportunity to comment about the objectives of the Society and how they relate to long-range research goals that are surfacing in genetics today.

Two of the four objectives of this Society are most pertinent to this discussion. Paraphrased these are 1) to promote basic and clinical research on diseases of the craniofacial complex, and 2) to apply these research results to the diagnosis and care of patients with craniofacial problems. The question that should be asked in regard to these objectives is ''how do they relate to the research trends in genetics during the past few years and in the future?'' Clearly, there has been a tremendous impact of the technology of molecular biology upon the study of heritable disorders in man. The use of recombinant DNA techniques and RFLP systems to detail man's genetic map has led to significant breakthroughs in the identification of both affected persons and those at risk for specified genetic diseases whose biologic mechanisms remain as yet undefined. Most notable of these diseases are Huntington disease, cystic fibrosis, and Duchenne muscular dystrophy. However, such spectacular advances in the description and classification of heritable disorders of the head and face have not occurred. Thus, the question facing our Society is, how can the objectives of this Society be amalgamated with the current emphasis on the application of molecular biology to the study of human genetics? One notable hindrance to the study of human clinical problems is the fact that there is a tremendous variation in clinical expression of monogenic traits such as seen in Crouzon disease or Treacher Collins syndrome. Furthermore, genetic heterogeneity is the key to understanding to-

Birth Defects: Original Article Series, Volume 25, Number 4, pages 3–5

day's clinical research effort. It should be obvious to us all that DNA studies and marker gene mapping tasks pursued at the present will ultimately resolve the question of genetic disease heterogeneity. It may take some time, but there is no question about the eventual outcome. However, the cost in time and money of such laboratory studies to evaluate individual patients on a routine basis is prohibitive. Research laboratories are spending millions of dollars attempting to locate genes that control specific traits on chromosomes. Thus, it seems apparent that there is a need for a rapid, simple, and inexpensive technique that will permit both the diagnosis of a given patient and the prognosis for his disease based upon those developmental mechanisms that have gone awry.

To those of us who work in the area of craniofacial dysmorphology it has long been apparent that many (perhaps even the majority) of the genetic syndromes have distinctive craniofacial characteristics. Unfortunately, variation in the clinical expression of a gene makes etiologic heterogeneity difficult to eliminate. If this latter problem can be resolved, the tools for study of craniofacial anomalies can be applied to an understanding of the developmental pathology involved. Once the dysmorphic mechanisms are understood, a rational basis for clinical treatment can be devised. Thus, it seems to me that it is not enough to know that a specific gene controlling a specific disease is located in a given chromosomal area. Even if the entire nucleotide sequence and the chromosomal location of a gene for a craniofacial disorder were known, this would not address the problem that the clinician sees or must deal with. There still remains a need for identification and description of disease pathogenesis and for an understanding of its relationship to the clinical problem. Only with such an understanding of gene expression and its relation to disease etiopathogenesis will it then become possible to provide comprehensive treatment and accurate genetic counseling. Thus, the clinical study of craniofacial dysmorphology, as promoted by the Society, is a valid and useful objective. We are steadily moving forward in this regard as evidenced by the subject material of previous Society programs.

It might be noted that clinicians have typically proceeded to develop methods of treatment for clinical disease long before a complete understanding of the disease process itself was ever elucidated. This is true today for heritable diseases affecting the craniofacial complex. However, this does not mean that we should relinquish our quest for an understanding of the basic dysmorphic processes, since only treatment based upon disease pathogenesis can provide the optimum result.

It is apparent to me that the objectives of this Society are no less valid today than when originally set down over 10 years ago. One important way in which molecular-clinical studies can complement each other lies in the area of confirmation. That is, a number of recent clinical research projects have been aimed at the identification of individuals who carry genes for a specific craniofacial trait but do not manifest them in a regular or consistent fashion. As we expand our knowledge of craniofacial dysmorphology and refine these identification criteria, it has become apparent that variable gene expression and genetic heterogeneity are two very difficult concepts to deal with for which molecular biology can provide the confirmation that we need. In my own research laboratory we have been employing the techniques of cephalometry and anthropometry to identify individuals who carry the X-linked gene for hypohidrotic ectodermal dysplasia. Statistically, we can identify these gene carrier individuals based upon morphometric features. However, the question remains as to the precision of the method. Now that the HED gene (or a closely linked marker gene) has been located on the X chromosome to pinpoint an affected individual, these same molecular techniques can now be used on the family members in which we have identified morphometric differences in order to validate the diagnosis. The morphometric approach, then, is basic science research aimed at identifying embryologic processes and even biochemical errors that define them. Morphometrics will not only provide the clinician with a blueprint of the dysmorphic anatomic processes that need correcting in order to achieve a harmonious result, but will also have the advantage of being relatively simple, rapid, and inexpensive to carry out. I hope that Society members will not feel "bypassed" by current emphasis on molecular research and will gain renewed zeal to pursue our Society objectives.

In conclusion, it is my opinion that there is still great need for an understanding of the dysmorphic mechanisms that occur in craniofacial syndromes, and the precision of molecular genetics can be used to validate and support the clinical research effort in this area.

Molecular Basis Among Hereditary Dentinal Defects: Pathobiology of Dentinal Phosphophoryn

John J. Sauk, DDS

Department of Pathology, Dental School, University of Maryland, Baltimore, MD 21201

There is increasing evidence that non-collagenous proteins associated with mineralized tissues play a critical role in the regulation of dentinogenesis. In an attempt to explain hereditary conditions that affect dentin and have no apparent manifestations in other mineralized tissues, those proteins that are unique to dentin were surveyed. A significant representative among the non-collagenous proteins of dentin is the acidic highly phosphorylated protein, "phosphophoryn" [1].

Dentinal phosphophoryns constitute one of the major soluble phosphoproteins of dentin that is obtained during demineralization of the tissues with EDTA [2]. These proteins are characterized by their high content of serine and aspartic acid. The seryl residues within the bovine molecule constitute approximately 545 residues/mol and are nearly completely phosphorylated. In addition, lysine, glycine, and glutamic acid are found in lesser amounts as well as a few residues of tyrosine and phenylalanine (Table 1) [3].

Historically, these dentinal proteins were difficult to characterize because of lability to mild acid and proteolytic enzymes. Also, the high charge density and heterogeneity in degree of phosphorylation made them difficult to purify [3]. These characteristics have resulted in controversy regarding their size and molecular weights. Currently, the bovine molecule has been regarded to have a molecular weight of 155,000 with the rat, rabbit, and human species having similar composition but varying in molecular mass (Table 2) [3].

The negative charge possessed by the phosphophoryns give this molecule a strong binding capacity for calcium ions. Structural studies have revealed

This work was supported by grants from the U.S. Public Health Service NIH, NIDR DE-08648, DE-07512.

Birth Defects: Original Article Series, Volume 25, Number 4, pages 7–13

TABLE 1. Amino Acid Composition of Bovine Dentin Phosphophoryn*

Residue	Residues/mol
Lys	45
His	6
Arg	3
Asp	452
Thr	8
Ser + Pse	545
Glu	14
Pro	6
Gly	27
Ala	7
1/2 Cys	1
Val	3
Met	1
Ile	3
Leu	4
Tyr	2
Phe	2
GIN	1
Total	1,130

*Stetler-Stevenson and Veis [3].

that at low calcium ion concentrations phosphophoryns fold back on themselves creating internally bridged structures, pleated sheets, while at high concentrations intermolecular aggregates are formed with calcium [4–7]. Phosphophoryns have been shown to accelerate formation of hydroxyapatite from solution when present at low concentrations [5,8,9], suggesting that they play some role in mineral nucleation and possibly in crystal growth [9].

Bovine phosphophoryn has been shown to bind to soluble collagen, to collagen fiber networks, and to gelatin gels but not to denatured collagen [10]. This interaction with collagen is primarily electrostatic and is influenced by ionic strength. Veis [11] has suggested that the binding of phosphophoryn to collagen fiber surfaces enhances the ability of dentin matrices to bind calcium via the conformational change seen on calcium binding [4,12] and thus strongly implicates these molecules in biological mineralization. A collagen-phosphophoryn conjugate has been described in dentinal matrices that has been exhaustively extracted with EDTA and digested with CNBr [7,10,13]. Studies conducted by Maier et al [14] have indicated that these conjugates probably form as late events and are temporally associated with passage of the mineralization front.

Developmental and biosynthetic studies reveal that phosphophoryns and

TABLE 2. Composition of Phosphophoryns From Various Species*

Amino Acid	Rabbit Incisor***	Rat incisor** α	Rat incisor** β	Fetal bovine molars‡	Human molars†
Asp	276	363	360	384	360
Thr	20	15	19	6	20
Ser + Pse	500	489	447	430	387
Glu	56	36	65	29	49
Pro	9	8.5	20	8	49
Gly	49	39	71	39	46
Ala	13	14	29	14	6.8
1/2 Cys		0.6			15
Val	5.3	2.4	6.7	7	8.5
Met		0.9	2.5		
Ill	4.0	2.5	4.4	6	3.6
Leu	5.9	2.4	5.7	8	8.2
Tyr	2.8	3.5	4.7	2	4.4
Phe	5.2	1.4	3.9	2	4.9
Lys	43	10.1	7.9	54	13.4
His	4.4	9.5	10.2	7	14.7
Arg	6.7	1.0	3.9	5	8.4

*Residues per 1,000 amino acid residues.
**Dimuzio and Veis [16].
***Richardson et al [24].
†Takagi et al [21].
‡Termine et al [25].

collagens reach their extracellular compartments by different routes [15,16]. Collagen is secreted from odontoblasts directly and makes up the bulk of predentin, while phosphophoryns are not found in predentin but are localized in either the odontoblast, Tomes process of the odontoblast, or within mineralized dentin [17]. Thus, phosphophoryns probably play their main role developmentally at the mineralization front rather than at premineralized sites. It is currently believed that these molecules have at least three potential roles in normal dentin: 1) transport of ions to the mineralization form, 2) localization of nucleation to specific regions of the collagen fiber surfaces, and 3) stabilization of the formed crystal [11].

Recently, Takagi and Sasaki [18] developed a histochemical technique based on the solubility of these proteins during demineralization (Table 3). In essence, teeth are treated with 0.5N acetic acid, which removes the mineral from teeth and leaves a number of the matrix proteins including phosphophoryns within the insoluble fraction. Frozen sections are then prepared and stained with Stains-all (Eastman Kodak Chem. Co.) to demonstrate the acidic proteins. For some studies teeth are demineralized in HCl to remove the

TABLE 3. Composition of Normal and DI Teeth*

Component	Normal	DI
Total organic matrix**	14.39	27.71
Protein contents***		
0.6 N HCl soluble	3.21	1.80
NaCi soluble	1.55	0.39
Insoluble residue	95.35	97.80
Phosphorous contents†		
Insoluble residue	0.050	0.004

*From Takagi et al [21].
**Percent of whole tooth, by weight.
***Percent of organic matrix, by weight.
†Percent of fraction, by weight. Phosphorus determined by the wet ash method of Kirkpatrick and Bishop.

majority of phosphophoryns, or ground undemineralized sections are prepared and the surfaces are etched with 0.5N acetic acid for 60 minutes prior to staining. Utilizing these techniques different morphological types of dentin can be identified microscopically. In so doing [18] it was revealed that phosphophoryn was found neither in predentin nor in mantel dentin. At high power, microscopic examination showed that phosphophoryn is present in the peritubular areas as well as in the intertubular regions of circumpulpal orthodentin but not in unmineralized interglobular dentin. Furthermore, phosphophoryn is not present in either secondary or reparative dentins.

Dentinogenesis imperfecta (DI), type II, is an autosomal dominant disorder of dentin. The teeth in this condition are characterized by their opalescence, marked attrition, and short roots constricted in the cervical regions. Also there is thickening of the bulk of dentin with obliteration of the pulp chambers. The dentin, though mineralized, has a low inorganic content when compared to normal teeth [19,20]. The collagen matrix appears to be normal but fails to mineralize completely. We have demonstrated biochemically that most of the non-collagenous proteins of dentin are either normal or present in higher amounts in this condition. Interestingly, these teeth lack phosphophoryns [21]. Utilizing the histochemical techniques described above, Takagi and Sasaki [18] also have supported these biochemical findings.

A clue to the molecular alteration in this hereditary condition derives from the histology of odontoblasts adjacent to various types of dentin (Table 4). Odontoblasts forming circumpulpal dentin are closely packed and have extended odontoblastic processes that are believed to be the delivery vehicle for phosphophoryns. In contrast, the odontoblastic processes of secondary, reparative, and mantel dentin are sparse or absent. Also, the mineralization front of these dentins contains matrix vesicles rather than phosphophoryn, which are thought to be the initiation site of mineralization [22,23]. Simi-

TABLE 4. Differences Among Various Types of Dentin*

	CD	MD	SD	RD	DI
Odontoblastic layer					
Intercellular spaces	−	+			+
Dentinal tubules					
Irregular arrangement	−		+	+	+
Reduction of no.	−	+	+	+	+
Collagen fibrils					
Coarse fibrils**	−	+	+		+
Matrix vesicles	−	+		+	
Hypomineralization	−	+	+	+	+
Phosphophoryn	+	−	−	−	−

*From Takagi and Sasaki [18].
**Coarse collagen fibrils arranged perpendicularly to the dentin surface. CD, circumpulpal dentin; MD, mantle dentin; SD, secondary dentin; RD, reparative dentin; DI, dentinogenesis imperfecta.

larly, in dentinogenesis imperfecta type II, odontoblasts that are separated from each other contain irregular and few odontoblastic processes and produce hypomineralized dentin (Table 4) [18]. These data indicate that complete differentiation of the odontoblast with formation of a Tomes process is an important mitigating factor in formation of highly mineralized circumpulpal dentin. Also, these findings demonstrate a close correlation between cell morphology and ensuing gene products, which typify a differentiated odontoblast. It is tempting to speculate that for this autosomal dominant condition (DI, type II) an alteration in a gene regulating phosphophoryn would account for the disorder. However, another consideration is that the alteration occurs at a level that affects differentiation with formation of the Tomes process. Thus, the phosphophoryn levels observed in DI might secondarily reflect the capable machinery available in an undifferentiated cell. Recent data demonstrating that integren receptors for various extracellular matrix proteins, i.e., fibronectin and laminin, can regulate differentiation in nerve cells [26], and endothelial cells [27] could place the gene defect for DI at a membrane receptor that controls the cytoskeletal organization of the odontoblastic process. In either case there appears to be a direct association between the presence of phosphophoryn and the development of a complete mineral phase. Clearly, further molecular studies are required for a better understanding of these dental conditions.

REFERENCES

1. Dimuzio MT, Veis A: Phosphophoryns—Major non-collagenous proteins of rat incisor dentin. Calcif Tissue Res 25:169–178, 1978.
2. Veis A, Spector AR, Zamoscianyk H: Isolation of an EDTA-soluble phosphoprotein from mineralizing bovine dentin. Biochim Biophys Acta 257:404–413, 1972.

3. Stetler-Stevenson WG, Veis A: Bovine dentin phosphophoryn: Composition and molecular weight. Biochemistry 22:4326–4335, 1983.
4. Lee SL, Veis A, Glonek T: Dentin phosphoprotein: An extracellular calcium-binding protein. Biochemistry 16:2971–2979, 1977.
5. Zanetti M, deBernard B, Jontell M, Linde A: Ca^{2+}-binding studies of the phosphoprotein from rat incisor dentine. Eur J Biochem 113:541–545, 1981.
6. Stetler-Stevenson WG: "Physical Characterization and Collagen Binding Properties of Bovine Dentin Phosphophoryn." PhD Dissertation. Evanston, IL: Northwestern University, 1983.
7. Curley-Joseph J, Veis A: The nature of covalent complexes of phosphoproteins with collagen in the bovine dentin matrix. J Dent Res 58:1625–1633, 1979.
8. Nawrot CF, Campbell DJ, Schroeder JK, Van Valkenburg M: Dental phosphoprotein-induced formation of hydroxyapatite during in vitro synthesis of amorphous calcium phosphate. Biochemistry 15:3445–3448, 1976.
9. Termine JD, Conn KM: Inhibition of apatite formation by phosphorylated metabolites and macromolecules. Calcif Tissue Res 22:149–157, 1976.
10. Dickson IR, Dimuzio MT, Volpin D, Ananthanarayanan S, Veis A: The extraction of phosphoproteins from bovine dentin. Calcif Tissue Res 19:51–61, 1975.
11. Veis A: Phosphoprotein of dentine and bone: Do they have a role in matrix mineralization. In Butler W (ed): "The Chemistry and Biology of Mineralized Tissues." Birmingham: Ebsco Media, 1984, pp 170–176.
12. Lee SL, Veis A: Cooperativity in calcium ion binding to repetitive carboxylate-serylphosphate polypeptides and the relationship of this property to dentin mineralization. Int J Pept Protein Res 16:231–240, 1980.
13. Lee SL, Veis A: Studies on the structure and chemistry of dentin collagen-phosphophoryn covalent complexes. Calcif Tissue Int 31:123–134, 1980.
14. Maier GD, Lechner JH, Veis A: The dynamics of formation of a collagen-phosphophoryn conjugate in relation to the passage of the mineralization front in rat incisor dentin. J Biol Chem 258:1450–1455, 1983.
15. Weinstock M, LeBlond CP: Radioautographic visualization of the deposition of a phosphoprotein at the mineralization front in the dentin of the rat incisor. J Cell Biol 56: 838–845, 1973.
16. Dimuzio MT, Veis A: The biosynthesis of phosphophoryns and dentin collagen in the continuously erupting rat incisor. J Biol Chem 253:6845–6852, 1978.
17. Veis A, Tsay T-G, Kanwat Y: An immunological study of the localization of dentin phosphophoryns in the tooth. In Ruch JV, Belcourt AB (eds): "Proceedings of the 2nd International Conference on Tooth Morphogenesis and Differentiation." Paris: INSERM Symposia Series, 1984, pp 223–232..
18. Takagi Y, Sasaki S: Histological distribution of phosphophoryn in normal and abnormal human dentins. J Oral Pathol 15:463–467, 1986.
19. Kerebel B, Daculsi G, Menanteau J, Kerebel LM: The inorganic phase in dentinogenesis imperfecta. J Dent Res 60:1655–1660, 1981.
20. Kirkpatrick DS, Bishop SH: Simplified wet ash procedure for total phosphorus analysis of organophosphonates in biological samples. Anal Chem 43:1707–1709, 1971.
21. Takagi Y, Veis A, Sauk JJ: Relation of mineralization defects in collagen matrices to non-collagenous protein components. Clin Orthop Rel Res 176:282–290, 1983.
22. Katchburian E: Membrane-bound bodies as initiators of mineralization of dentine. J Anat 116:285–302, 1974.

23. Hirschfield Z, Bab I, Tamari I, Sela J: Primary mineralization of dentin in rats after pulp capping with calcium-hydroxide. J Oral Pathol 11:426–431, 1982.
24. Richardson WS, Beegle WF, Butler WT, Munksgaard EC: The phosphoprotein of rabbit incisors. J Dent Res 56:233–237, 1977.
25. Termine JD, Belcourt AB, Miyamoto MS, Conn KM: Properties of dissociatively extracted fetal tooth matrix proteins. II. Separation and purification of fetal bovine dentin phosphoprotein. J Biol Chem 255:9769–9772, 1980.
26. Dodd J, Jessell TM: Axon guidance and patterning of neuronal projections in vertebrates. Science 242:692–699, 1988.
27. Kubota Y, Kleinman HK, Martin GR, Lawley TJ: Role of laminin and basement membrane in the morphological differentiation of human endothelial cells into capillary-like structures. J Cell Biol 1589–1598, 1988.

Mast Cells in Bone Remodeling: Using a Genetically Defined Mouse Model as a Clue to Human Disease

Robyn Rosenstein, DDS, Gary Greenberg, PhD, Michael Melnick, DDS, PhD, and Cedric Minkin, PhD

Department of Basic Sciences and Graduate Program in Craniofacial Biology, School of Dentistry, University of Southern California, Los Angeles, CA 90089-0641

Mastocytosis is the proliferation of mast cells in viscera and other tissues. It is a multiorgan disease that most commonly affects the skin and skeletal system. Over 70% of patients with systemic mastocytosis demonstrate radiographically detectable bone lesions [1–3]. The bone lesions may be unifocal, multifocal, or diffuse and may be of the osteosclerotic or osteoporotic type or mixed [4,5].

Although familial cases have been reported, systemic mastocytosis occurs most frequently as an isolated event. Among patients who develop mastocytosis during childhood, the mean age of onset is under 1 year. The disease occurs equally in both sexes, and all races are affected. Identical twins with mastocytosis have been reported, as have cases where the disease involves one identical twin [6,7]. Based on over 47 familial cases reported in the literature, the pattern of inheritance is thought to be autosomal dominant [8].

Given the clinical picture of generalized bone disease, there are two possibilities: 1) the bone lesions are secondary to the mast cell proliferation, because mast cells play a role in bone remodeling; or 2) the bone lesions are a pleiotropic manifestation of the mutant gene, and mast cells have nothing to do with the lesions observed, because mast cells do not play a role in bone remodeling.

In order to begin to address these two alternative hypotheses, we chose to investigate the role of mast cells in bone remodeling by using a mouse mutant that is deficient in mast cells.

This work was supported by NIH grants DE-07225 to G.G., DE-04961 to C.M., DE-07006 to M.M., and the Boone Chair Fund.

Birth Defects: Original Article Series, Volume 25, Number 4, pages 15–25

Mast cell-deficient mice differ from the wild type at the W locus, located on chromosome 5 [9]. From a cross between the W/+ and Wv/+, we use the +/+ genotype (wild type), and the W/Wv genotype (mast cell-deficient mutant). The W/+ and Wv/+ show only a slight decrease in mast cells. The W/Wv mice have virtually no detectable mast cells, have macrocytic anemia, and lack melanocytes [10,11]. The mast cell and erythrocyte cell populations can be reconstituted by bone marrow transplants from the normal +/+ mouse [12,13]. Thus, the genetically mast cell-deficient mouse together with its normal littermate provide a unique opportunity to compare the expression of a biologic response (e.g., bone remodeling), in vivo, in the presence and absence of mast cells [14].

The bone remodeling cycle is a sequence of interrelated actions of the various bone cell types resulting first in the removal, and then the replacement of a quantum of bone [15]. Perturbation of a specific site of resting bone results in activation of precursors leading to osteoclastic resorption, which is then coupled in the reversal phase to a subsequent active wave of bone formation. In this, a cycle of bone remodeling is completed [16–19].

Tran Van et al have developed an experimental model in which bone remodeling is induced in the mandibular buccal periosteum of rats [20]. Extraction of the upper molars results in hypereruption (egression) of the mandibular molars owing to the lack of opposing occlusion. This perturbation of a normal occlusal relationship induces a synchronous and reproducible cycle of bone remodeling activity on the mandibular buccal periosteal surface, which can be quantitated using standard histomorphometric technique. Using this approach in rats, both the time of onset and duration of each phase of the bone remodeling cycle has been quantitated, and the effects of various physiologic variables have been studied [21,22].

Our null hypothesis was that there would be no difference in the bone remodeling activity of the mast cell-sufficient and mast cell-deficient mouse.

MATERIALS AND METHODS

The specific design of this investigation involved extracting the upper row of molars on the right side in 20 adult (age 4–5 months) +/+ and W/Wv mice. Control specimens were obtained from the left side mandible at day 0. Mandibles were collected after intracardiac glutaraldehyde perfusion fixation at days 0 (day of extraction), 1, 2, 3, 4, 5, 6, 7, 10, and 16. Tissues were prepared for light microscopy and electron microscopy, with emphasis on maximizing high-quality preservation of cellular integrity [23,24]. Tissues were embedded in Epon, and thin and ultrathin sections were cut parallel to the occlusal plane. Nine samples were taken for each animal, three samples at each of three sample sites located at the upper, middle, and lower regions of the top 270 μm of crestal bone. The upper site is defined as the first 90 μm of continuous periosteum beginning from the most crestal alveolar bone, the middle site is the next 90 μm, and the lower site is 180–270 μm from the top crestal bone. Microanatomical landmarks confirmed the reproducibility of sample site from animal to animal.

Histomorphometry was performed on all nine samples for each animal. Measurements were taken adjacent to the first and second molars. Periosteal surfaces with the following cell types and characteristics were measured: 1) intermediate osteoblasts, 2) flattened osteoblasts, 3) Howship's lacunae with osteoclasts, 4) Howship's lacunae without osteoclasts or osteoid, 5) Howship's lacunae with osteoblasts and osteoid, and 6) cuboidal osteoblasts (see Fig. 1). In addition, maximum mean wall thickness was measured from the last cement line [25]. Paper tracings of these areas noting the various cell types were prepared using high magnification (×63 planapo lens) on 1 μm sections with a micrometer eyepiece and a drawing tube extension. The percentage of periosteal surface occupied by various cell types was calculated from the paper tracings using a digitizing tablet and Sigma Scan computer software (Jandel Scientific; Sausalito, CA) (Fig. 1).

Parfitt et al, Eriksen, and others have established functional relationships with the cell morphologies listed. For example, double staining (fluorescent and brightfield) has shown that appositional rates of osteoid are greatest for cuboidal osteoblasts and lowest for flat osteoblasts [26,27]. Further, cell types are associated with successive stages in the bone remodeling cycle. Quiescent surfaces are characterized by intermediate osteoblasts. Activation is associated with flattened osteoblasts and the arrival of osteoclast precursors at or near the periosteal surface. Resorbing surfaces are defined by osteoclasts in Howship's lacunae, and reversal surfaces are defined by Howship's lacunae without osteoclasts or osteoid. Cuboidal osteoblasts and Howship's lacunae containing osteoblasts and osteoid are defined as active forming surfaces [28].

Statistical analysis of percentage data, which is not normally distributed, required arcsin transformation. A nested ANOVA revealed that it was appropriate to average the three samples within a given sample site. Using these averages, a series of three way ANOVAs was conducted to examine interactions between percentage of periosteal surface covered by different cell types, post-extraction day, sample site, and genotype.

RESULTS

Variation of the periosteal surface covered by different cell types (i.e., osteoblasts, Howship's lacunae with osteoclasts, and Howship's lacunae without osteoclasts or osteoid tissue) was evaluated with respect to post-

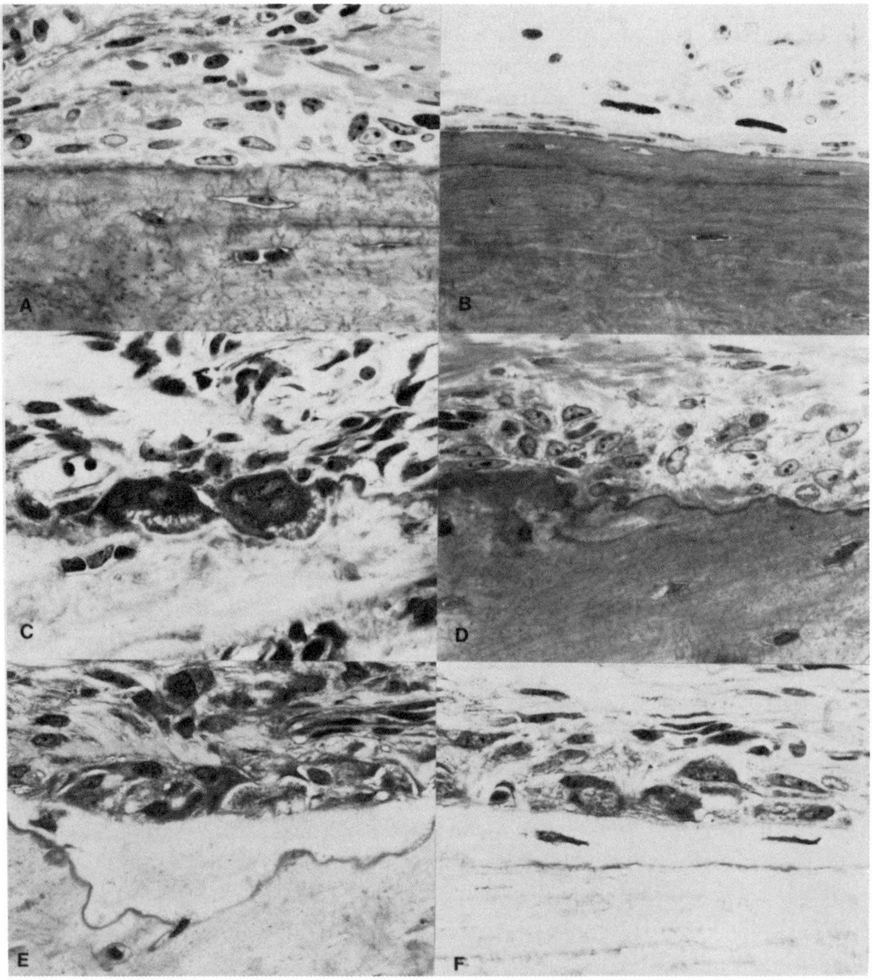

Fig. 1. Photomicrographs illustrating characteristic cell surfaces used in histomorphometric analysis of bone remodeling. **(A)** Intermediate osteoblasts. **(B)** Flattened osteoblasts. **(C)** Howship's lacunae with osteoclasts. **(D)** Howship's lacunae without osteoclasts or osteoid tissue. **(E)** Howship's lacunae with osteoblasts and osteoid tissue. **(F)** Cuboidal osteoblasts. Modified paragon stain. ×1000.

extraction day and genotype, at each sample site. The results of this ANOVA are shown in Table 1. Cell type shows a significant interaction by post-extraction day, but not genotype. Thus, the space occupied by various cell types found along the mandibular periosteal surface is dependent upon the

TABLE 1. F-Tests of Significance for All Cell Types†

Interactions	Upper	Middle	Lower
Cell type × day	2.26*	2.72**	1.24
Cell type × genotype	0.71	0.47	0.69
Day × genotype	0.01	0.03	0.02

†Results of analysis of variance at each sample site. See text for details.
$^{*}P < .05$
$^{**}P < .01$

time lapsed following extraction of the upper molars. The strongest interaction between cell type and post-extraction day is at the middle sample site, while the lower site showed no significant interaction. Distribution of the periosteal surface covered by different cell types included in the first analysis are graphically represented by their associated functional phases of bone remodeling activity in the +/+ mouse (Fig. 2). Here it can be seen that resorption is at its maximum at day 2, reversal is at day 3, and formation, after remodeling is induced, dominates from day 5 post-extraction (Fig. 2; Table 1).

An additional analysis of variance was designed to evaluate the variation of periosteal surface covered by osteoblast cell types specifically, since distinctive osteoblast morphologies represent different functions and appear to produce bone matrix at different appositional rates. The osteoblast cell type analysis included intermediate, flattened, cuboidal, and Howship's lacunae with osteoblasts and osteoid tissue. The results presented in Table 2 show a significant interaction for both osteoblast cell type by post-extraction day and osteoblast cell type by genotype at the middle sample site. Thus, the space occupied by various osteoblast cell types along the periosteal surface is dependent upon the time lapsed following extraction of the upper molars and the genotype. Analysis of actively forming surfaces (Howship's lacunae with osteoblasts and osteoid tissue, and cuboidal osteoblasts) showed a significant post-extraction day by genotype interaction (Table 3). Distribution of the periosteal surface covered by different active bone-forming cells for both genotypes is shown graphically in Figure 3. It can be seen that active bone-forming cells appear in the +/+ mouse several days before the W/Wv mouse (Fig. 3; Table 3).

Having established a difference between the two strains of mice for bone-forming surfaces, we evaluated the maximum mean wall thickness from the last cement line, as a measure of osteoblast activity. There were significant differences among sites and among days but not among genotypes; there was a significant interaction between genotype and post-extraction day (Table 4).

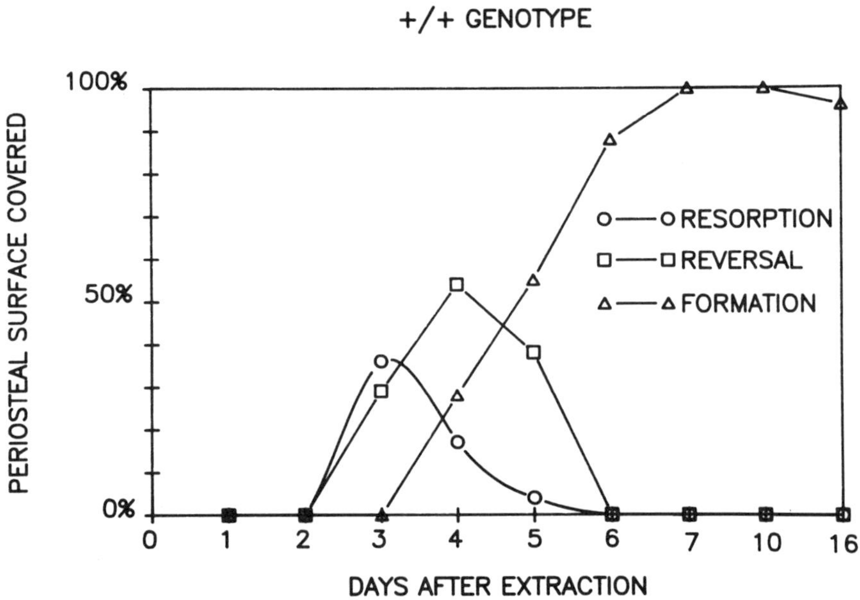

Fig. 2. Sequence of bone remodeling in normal (+/+ genotype) mice observed at the middle sample site following experimental induction. Phases of the remodeling cycle are represented by the following cell types: Resorption, by Howship's lacunae with osteoclasts; reversal, by Howship's lacunae without osteoclasts or osteoid tissue; and formation, by intermediate, flattened, cuboidal osteoblasts and Howship's lacunae with osteoblasts and osteoid tissue.

TABLE 2. F-Tests of Significance for Osteoblast Cell Types†

Interactions	Upper	Middle	Lower
Cell type × day	2.83*	3.42**	2.14
Cell type × genotype	1.96	4.74*	1.55
Day × genotype	0.07	0.04	0.02

†Results of analysis of variance at each sample site. See text for details.
*$P < .05$
**$P < .01$

This indicates that the amount of osteoid matrix formed by each of the two strains of mice differs for any given post-experimental day. Further, the +/+ mouse demonstrated a greater mean wall thickness at the termination of the experiment than did the mast cell-deficient W/Wv mouse (Table 4).

DISCUSSION

These preliminary findings, involving variation in periosteal surface covered by different functional cell types and matrix production, indicate that

TABLE 3. F-Tests of Significance for Forming Surfaces

Source of variance	df	F-value
Sample site	2	24.8**
Day post-extraction	9	39.2**
Genotype	1	10.2**
Site × day	18	1.7
Site × genotype	2	0.5
Day × genotype	9	3.0*

*$P < .05$
**$P < .01$

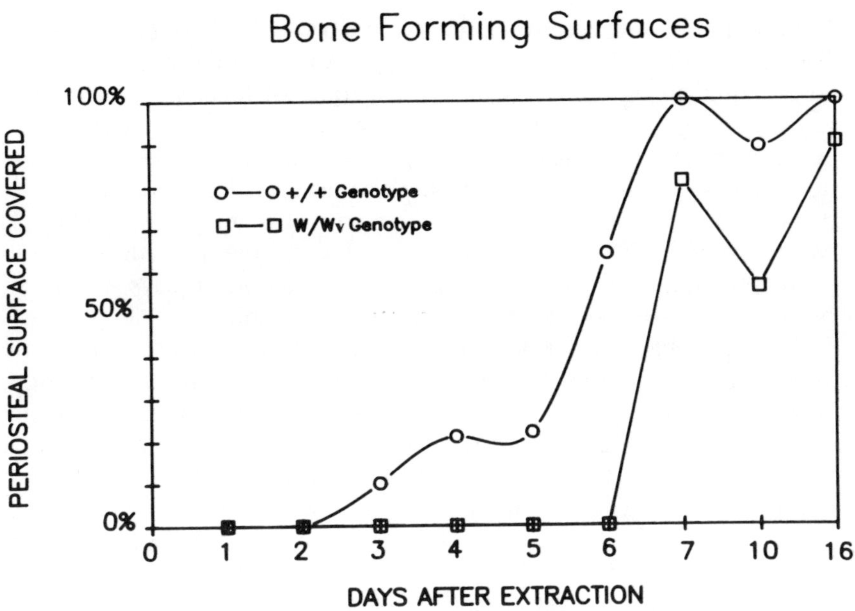

Fig. 3. Comparison of active bone formation phase of bone remodeling between normal (+/+) and mutant (W/Wv) mice.

there are differences between genotypes. Consequently, we can reject our null hypothesis that there are no differences in the bone remodeling activity of the mast cell-sufficient and mast cell-deficient mouse.

Distinct and significant phases of cellular activity throughout the experimental time period define the cellular kinetics of a single bone remodeling cycle in the two strains of mice used in these experiments. These data are consistent with those reported for the rat and confirm the sequential and reproducible stimulation of the remodeling cycle using this egression model in the mouse.

TABLE 4. F-Tests of Significance for Mean Wall Thickness

Source of Variance	df	F-value
Sample site	2	15.2**
Day post-extraction	9	18.9**
Genotype	1	2.1
Site × day	18	2.1
Site × genotype	2	0
Day × genotype	9	2.9*

*$P < .05$
**$P < .01$

The differences found between the two genotypes were significant at the middle sample site. This illustrates the importance of a defined sample site when utilizing the egression model as a method of inducing synchronous bone remodeling. The critical region (of mandibular crestal periosteum) to examine for bone remodeling in this mouse tooth egression model is approximately 90–180 μm down (apical) from the most crestal periosteum. This is a region that is typically quiescent in an animal with normal occlusion. However, when occlusion is disrupted by the extraction procedure used in this experiment, then accurate sampling of this area over 16 days will reveal each phase of the remodeling cycle, including activation.

As far as the phases of the bone remodeling cycle are concerned, there are significant differences between the normal and mast cell-deficient mutant in the response of bone-forming cells to the induction of a bone-remodeling cycle. The W/Wv mouse was slower to begin remodeling, trailed several days behind the +/+ mouse, and spent less time in the formation portion of the cycle (Fig. 3). Thus, in the absence of mast cells there is a slower response to activation of bone formation and a decrease in the overall amount of bone matrix formed.

Our results, obtained in the absence of mast cells in the W/Wv mouse, are complimentary to human studies of mastocytosis patients with excessive numbers of mast cells. In an evaluation of trabecular bone from transiliac crest biopsies in patients with systemic mastocytosis, Fallon et al presented evidence of an abnormal accumulation of osteoid, peritrabecular fibrosis and increased numbers of osteoblasts and osteoclasts. They concluded that these patients experienced accelerated bone remodeling [29].

It is appreciated in bone physiology that the local elaboration of regulatory molecules significantly influences the cellular events in bone remodeling [30–34]. Included in these regulatory molecules are autocrine and paracrine molecules such as cytokines, growth factors, and prostaglandins. The presence of mast cells may act to modulate local factors, which could potentiate or inhibit various regulatory mechanisms.

Mast cells contain granules of biologically active substances, which include various enzymes, chemotactic peptides, histamine, proteoglycan heparin, and other regulatory molecules [35,36]. It has been shown that aside from the massive degranulation associated with an IgE-mediated response, that cell-cell contacts and transfer of mast cell contents can occur [37]. Thus, they have the potential to modulate the microenvironment [38,39]. Furthermore, mast cells may also effect local cell kinetics. Norrby et al have shown that mesenchymal cell proliferation increases significantly in response to a product(s) secreted by mast cells [40–42]. Hatanaka et al also demonstrated the mitogenic effect of mast cells on local cell populations in the wild-type mouse (+/+) relative to the mast cell-deficient mouse (W/Wv) [42].

In conclusion, our results, taken together with those of human studies, suggest that mast cells play a role in bone remodeling. With respect to the bone lesions observed in systemic mastocytosis, it is reasonable to assume that the increased numbers and activity of mast cells cause a cellular proliferation that results in either osteolytic or osteogenic skeletal pathology depending upon the bone surface and cell types affected. The differences observed in the present studies with mast cell-deficient mutants further reveal that although bone remodeling can proceed in the absence of mast cells, it proceeds somewhat slower. This suggests that the local modulatory role of mast cells is not a limiting factor in bone remodeling but may be important only as a supplementary mechanism or in pathologic conditions. This suggestion is being examined with additional experiments using the tooth egression model and may be further tested by examining experimental models where the perturbation of the bone remodeling cycle is more extreme than the physiologic perturbation caused by tooth egression.

ACKNOWLEDGMENTS

We acknowledge the following colleagues for their invaluable advice, support, and assistance: Drs. Roland Baron, Ken Byrd, Helen Gruber, and Pablo Bringas.

REFERENCES

1. Rafii M, Firooznia H, Golimbu C, Balthazar E: Pathologic fracture in systemic mastocytosis: Radiographic spectrum and review of the literature. Clin Orthop 180:260–267, 1983.
2. Harvard CW, Scott RB: Urticaria pigmentosa with visceral and skeletal lesions. Q J Med 28:459–470, 1959.
3. Sagher F, Cohen C, Schorr S: Concomitant bone changes in urticaria pigmentosa. J Invest Dermatol 18:425–432, 1952.
4. Rosenbaum RC, Frieri M, Metcalfe DD: Patterns of skeletal scintigraphy and their rela-

tionship to plasma and urinary histamine levels in systemic mastocytosis. J Nucl Med 25:859–864, 1984.
5. Lucaya J, Perez-Candela V, Aso C, Clavo J: Mastocytosis with skeletal and gastrointestinal involvement in infancy: Two case reports and a review of the literature. Radiology 131:363–366, 1979.
6. Stein DH: Mastocytosis: A review. Pediatr Dermatol 3:365–375, 1986.
7. Fowler JF, Parsley WM, Cotter PG: Familial urticaria pigmentosa. Arch Dermatol 122: 80,81, 1986.
8. McKusick VA: "Mendelian Inheritance in Man: Catalogs of Autosomal Dominant, Autosomal Recessive, and x-Linked Phenotypes," 7th Edition. Baltimore and London: The Johns Hopkins University Press, 1986, p 481.
9. Russell ES: Hereditary anemias of the mouse: A review for geneticists. Adv Genet 20: 357–459, 1979.
10. Bernstein S, Russell ES: Implantation of normal blood forming tissue in genetically anemic mice without X-irradiation. Proc Soc Exp Biol Med 101:769–773, 1959.
11. Ponvert C, Galoppin L, Scheinmann P, Canu P, Burtin C: Tissue histamine levels in male and female mast cell deficient mice (W/Wv) and in their littermates (Wv/+, W/+ and +/+). Agents Actions 17:1–4, 1985.
12. Sharkis SJ, Wiktor-Jedrzejczak W, Ahmed A, Santos GW, McKee A, Sell KW: Antitheta-sensitive regulatory cell (TSRC) and hematopoiesis: Regulation of differentiation of transplanted stem cells in W/Wv anemic and normal mice. Blood 52:802–817, 1978.
13. Kitamura Y, Go S, Hatanaka K: Decrease of mast cells in W/Wv mice and their increase by bone marrow transplantation. Blood 52:447–452, 1978.
14. Galli SJ, Kitamura Y: Genetically mast-cell-deficient W/Wv and Sl/Sld mice: Their value for the analysis of the roles of mast cells in biologic responses in vitro. Am J Pathol 127:191–198, 1987.
15. Baron R, Vignery A, Horowitz M: Lymphocytes, macrophages and the regulation of bone remodeling. In Peck WA (ed): "Bone Min Res, Annual 2." Amsterdam: Elsevier Science Publishers B.V., 1983, pp 175–243.
16. Jaworski ZFG: Coupling of bone formation to bone resorption. Calcif Tissue Int 36: 531–535, 1984.
17. Meunier PJ: Cellular mechanisms of bone remodeling evaluated at the intermediary level of organization of bone. Adv Exp Med Biol 208:247–254, 1986.
18. Peck WA, Rifas L, Cheng SL, Shen V: The local regulation of bone remodeling. Adv Exp Med Biol 208:255–259, 1986.
19. Parfitt AM: The cellular basis of bone remodeling: The quantum concept reexamined in light of recent advances in the cell biology of bone. Calcif Tissue Int 36:S37–S45, 1984.
20. Tran Van P, Vignery A, Baron R: Cellular kinetics of the bone remodeling sequence in the rat. Anat Rec 202:445–451, 1982.
21. Klapisz-Wolikow M, Saffar JL: Etude d'une sequence de remaniement experimental induite sur le perioste mandibulaire du rat. J Biol Buccale 14:263–271, 1986.
22. Saffar JL, Leroux P: Role of prostaglandins in bone resorption in a synchronized remodeling sequence in the rat. Bone 9:141–145, 1988.
23. Cole AA, Walters LM: Tartrate-resistant acid phosphatase in bone and cartilage following decalcification and cold-embedding in plastic. J Histochem Cytochem 35:203–206, 1987.
24. Baron R, Neff L, Tran Van P, Nefussi JR, Vignery A: Kinetic and cytochemical identification of osteoclast precursors and their differentiation into multinucleated osteoclasts. Am J Pathol 122:363–378, 1986.
25. Villanueva AR, Kujawa M, Mathews CHE, Parfitt AM: Identification of the mineraliza-

tion front: Comparison of a modified toluidine blue stain with tetracycline fluorescence. Metab Bone Dis Rel Res 5:41–45, 1983.
26. Parfitt AM, Villanueva AR, Crouch MM, Mathews CHE, Duncan H: Classification of osteoid seams by combined use of cell morphology and tetracycline labelling. Evidence for intermittency of mineralization. In Meunier PJ (ed): ''Bone Histomorphometry,'' 2nd International Workshop, Lyon, 1976. Lyon: Societé de la Nouvelle Imprimerie Fournie, 1977, pp 299–310.
27. Eriksen EF: Normal and pathological remodeling of human trabecular bone: Three dimensional reconstruction of the remodeling sequence in normals and in metabolic bone disease. Endocr Rev 7:379–408, 1986.
28. Parfitt AM, Villanueva AR, Mathews CHE, Aswani SA: Kinetics of matrix and mineral apposition in osteoporosis and renal osteodystrophy. Relationship to rate of turnover and to cell morphology. Metab Bone Dis Rel Res 2S:213–219, 1980.
29. Fallon MD, Whyte MP, Teitelbaum SL: Systemic mastocytosis associated with generalized osteopenia: Histopathological characterization of the skeletal lesion using undecalcified bone from two patients. Hum Pathol 12:813–820, 1981.
30. Raisz LG, Kream BE: Regulation of bone formation. N Engl J Med 309:29–35, 83–89, 1983.
31. Canalis E: The hormonal and local regulation of bone formulation. Endocr Rev 4:62–67, 1983.
32. Ibbotson KJ, D'Souza SM, Kanis JA, Douglas DL, Russell RGG: Physiological and pharmacological regulation of bone resorption. Metab Bone Dis Rel Res 2:177–189, 1980.
33. Gowen M, MacDonald BR, Hughes DE, Skjodt H, Russell RGG: Immune cells and bone resorption. Adv Exp Med Biol 208:261–273, 1986.
34. Urist MR, DeLange RJ, Finerman GAM: Bone cell differentiation and growth factors. Science 220:680–686, 1983.
35. Schwartz LB: Mediators of human mast cells and human mast cell subsets. Ann Allergy 58:226–237, 1987.
36. Lewis RA, Austen KF: Mediation of local homeostasis and inflammation by leukotrienes and other mast cell-dependent compounds. Naturre 293:103–108, 1981.
37. Greenberg G, Burnstock G: A novel cell-to-cell interaction between mast cells and other cell types. Exp Cell Res 147:1–13, 1983.
38. Azizkhan RG, Azizkhan JC, Clifford J, Zetter BR, Folkman J: Mast cell heparin stimulates migration of capillary endothelial cells in vitro. J Exp Med 152:931–944, 1980.
39. Yoffe JR, Taylor DJ, Woolley DE: Mast-cell products and heparin stimulate the production of mononuclear-cell factor by cultured human monocyte/macrophages. Biochem J 230:83–88, 1985.
40. Norrby K, Enerback L, Franzen L: Mast cell activation and tissue cell proliferation. Cell Tissue Res 170:289–303, 1978.
41. Norrby K: On the 48/80-induced secretion of tissue mast cells and its mitogenic effect on nearby cells in the intact rat. Virchows Arch [B] 38:57–65, 1981.
42. Hatanaka K, Imakita M, Go S, Yamamoto A: Effects of degranulation of mast cells on proliferation of mesenchymal cells in the mesentery of mice. Cell Tissue Res 246:53–56, 1986.

Terminology of Craniofacial Anomalies

John M. Opitz, MD

Department of Medical Genetics, Shodair Children's Hospital, Helena, MT 59601

INTRODUCTION

In 1895 Wilhelm His [1] edited the first edition of "Nomina Anatomica" (Anatomical Nomenclature). Since that time many efforts have been made at defining terms dealing with the normal and abnormal developmental attributes of human structure [2,3]. Correct terminology representing a consensus of workers in the field is an undoubted aid to understanding and to communicating facts and interpretations to patients, colleagues, and oneself. Consistency in use does not necessarily guarantee correctness and it does not obviate the need to change, as additional understanding leads to greater complexity of the subject and the need to create hierarchical subheadings under the more general, formerly employed, term.

In his book "Natural Inheritance" (1889) Francis Galton [4] detailed the methods of quantitative human genetics (Galtonian inheritance as opposed to Mendelian inheritance). In the analysis of normal (continuous) variability, he introduced exact, anthropometric, and statistical approaches and methods that have become standard in the field and have over the past century served to document the fact that normality is infinitely more variable than abnormality. It is as important to distinguish between the philtrum and the upper lip as it is to distinquish between the five major classes of developmental abnormalities of the external ear, namely, abnormalities of migration, differentiation, rotation, folding, and growth. Abnormalities of forward rotation are viewed clinically as abnormalities of posterior angulation, and the assessment of "low-set ears" in clinical practice continues to be beset with difficulties.

In a larger sense, this discussion pertains to the developmental aspects of

This work was supported in part by a grant from the Montana Department of Health and Environmental Sciences under HB716.

Birth Defects: Original Article Series, Volume 25, Number 4, pages 27–37

the concepts of dysplasia, malformation, and deformity, and to syndromes as contrasted to complex monotopic or polytopic developmental fields.

The discussion also briefly alludes to the three cardinal epistemologic attributes of malformations in general, including the presence/absence as attribute of causality, variability as attribute of pathogenesis, and the attribute of phylogeneity that stresses the need to view malformations in all cases in their evolutionary perspective, since it is evident that the genetic changes responsible for phylogenetic changes withing the phylum also play a role in normal ontogeny.

Going in a caudal direction along the neuraxis, metamerism first becomes apparent in the occipital region. Whether the more rostral portions of neuraxial structures represent a complex evolutionary fusion product of several cranial metameres, or "vertebrae," was the subject of heated debate in the 19th century; it was begun by Johann Wolfgang von Goethe and remains unresolved. The complexity of developmental abnormalities that may occur in the metameric and apparently non-metameric portions of the head is so bewildering that it would seem foolhardy to attempt to order them according to developmental principles. Nevertheless, it is possible with careful attention to anatomy, embryology, and comparative aspects, to group most craniofacial anomalies under a few headings, keeping in mind some of the unusual developmental attributes that set craniofacial structure apart from trunk and limbs; here, I refer primarily to the extremely important role of the cranial neural crest in normal craniofacial morphogenesis.

DYSPLASIAS

The International Working Group (IWG) [2] defined a dysplasia as an abnormality of cellular or tissue differentiation, i.e., as a "dyshistogenesis" usually arising after organogenesis.

It is a fundamental axiom of developmental analysis "dass Form vor der Structur entsteht" as Meckel apparently put it early in the 19th century, i.e., that organogenesis precedes histogenesis. Thus, while the organogenetic events during embryogenesis involve cells, it is not the later, organ-specific histologic attributes of these cells that are the critical factor in organogenesis; rather, they are the tissue non-specific but organ-specific morphogenetic interaction of these cells with each other in compartmentalized groups according to specific biochemical and biophysical means that characterizes the initial stages of morphogenesis. A common sense confirmation from clinical practice of this dictum is the fact that most malformed organs are not histologically abnormal or highly predisposed to the development of cancers and that most cancers do not arise in malformed organs. The three organs in which there is an exception to this rule in the sense that histogenesis is a major contributor to morphogenesis, namely the brain, kidneys, and lungs, are also the three organs with the highest incidence of dysplasias, i.e., abnormalities of tissue or histologic differentiation. These are all organs in which histogenetic morphogenesis continues right through fetal life and, in certain respects, after birth.

However, for our purposes it suffices to recall that most craniofacial malformations are not stigmatized by gross histologic abnormalities except for certain interesting exceptions.

The reason it may be appropriate to invoke the concept of dysplasia in analyzing craniofacial anomalies is that cranial neural crest plays such an important role in the development of the head [5,6], and, since it is a tissue, the question arises whether a malformation complex, such as mandibulofacial dysostosis or the craniofacial anomalies of the Accutane disruption sequence, ought not to be called a dysplasia. After all, there exists precedence in speaking of hip "dysplasia." However, in that case acetabular "hypoplasia" seems to be a more correct designation. A presumption of skeletal "dysplasia" is undocumented in many cases since the bones of such patients appear histologically normal in postnatal life. Numerous CNS dysplasias are known, and renal nephroblastomatosis and the pulmonary lesions of tuberous sclerosis are additional examples of dysplasias in other organs. Some of these abnormalities are hamartomas consisting of an abnormal composition, proportion, and frequently location of histologically normal cells. Thus, the production of normal cells does not necessarily guarantee normal differentiation, and it is rather the determinant aspects of the cells during early morphogenesis that are of importance to us rather than the later abnormalities of histogenesis. Thus, cranial neural crest cells appear to have an extremely important determinative function in the sequence of morphogenetic events that leads to normal craniofacial structure; indeed, they have been demonstrated to participate actively in the morphogenesis of these structures in regions as far "south" as the heart.

Where dysplasias are abnormalities of histogenesis, *malformations* are abnormalities of organogenesis. A *primary* malformation represents an intrinsic abnormality *of* a developmental field; a *secondary* malformation (or disruption) represents an extrinsic abnormality *in* a developmental field.

Developmental fields are the morphogenetically reactive units of the embryo that effect organogenesis in a spatially and temporally coordinated and epimorphically hierarchical manner through processes of determination, induction, and differentiation [7,8].

Nevertheless, neural crest dysplasias exist and have been summed by Robert Bolande and Malcolm Johnston under the heading of the "neurocristopathies" [9,10]. In such cases as the Waardenburg syndrome with megacolon and piebaldism [11], these dysplasias include congenital megacolon with hypoganglionosis, hyperganglionosis, and ectopic ganglia in the lamina propria. The neurocristopathies also include such tumors as schwannomas, carotid body tumors, and pheochromocytomas. On the basis of numerous clinical observations, teratologic studies, animal data, and insights from experimental embryology, we conclude that the morphogenetic activities of neural crest cells can be disturbed to produce the malformation complexes mandibulofacial dysostosis, otocephaly, and the DiGeorge complex. Examples include the *oel* mouse [12–14], hypervitaminosis A [15,16], the fetal alcohol syndrome, and the Accutane syndrome (or disruption sequence) [17] presented before us in the past by Drs. Johnston and Sulik [18] and Lammer, among many others.

However, there are rare occasions in which dysplasias do interfere with craniofacial morphogenesis. The best known are epignathus or dermoids with teratomatous disruption, which are better and more commonly documented elsewhere in the body as in the so-called Currarino triad of sacrococcygeal teratoma with anterior sacral meningocele, developmental abnormality of sacrum, anus, and caudal portions of spinal cord [19].

An exceptionally nice illustration of a dysplasia malformation syndrome is the entity described by Penchaszadeh et al [20] when Victor Penchaszadeh was still working in Venezuela. This was a new autosomal dominant disorder seen in eight individuals in three generations of a Venezuelan family characterized by congenital symmetrical upper lid and naso-palpebral lipomas, bilateral symmetrical upper and lower palpebral colobomas located at the junction of the inner and middle thirds of the lids, telecanthus, maxillary hypoplasia, broad forehead, widow's peak, abnormal pattern of eyebrows and eyelashes, and maldevelopment of the lacrimal puncta. The authors postulated that the primary defect could involve a dysplasia of adipose tissue leading to naso-palpebral and upper lid lipomas during embryogenesis, with the rest of the malformations being secondary to interference of morphogenesis of the mid-upper face developmental field from the lipomatous hamartomas. As an alternate hypothesis the authors postulate a central rather than a peripheral mechanism of malformation involving defective migration or differentiation of neural crest cells. with the application of monoclonal antibodies, major advances have been made in the study of the morphogenetic role of cranial neural crest [21] and especially of the function of laminin in these complex processes [22].

MINOR ANOMALIES

Most of the minor anomalies that we encounter daily in clinical genetics involve craniofacial structures. They include hypo- and hypertelorism, posterior angulation of auricles, long/short ears, short palpebral fissures, long upper lip, and epicanthic folds correlated with less mature than normal (or flatter) bridge of nose.

These minor anomalies are abnormalities of phenogenesis, i.e., the period of morphogenesis after completion of organogenesis at the end of the 8th/beginning of the 9th week of prenatal life [23]. Although some, such as epicanthic folds, do not appear to have a quantitative correlate, most of the anomalies listed above are quantitative abnormalities of morphogenesis subsumed by human geneticists and anthropologists with anthropometric and quantitative radiologic studies in the form of hundreds of distribution curves, not always with a normal or Gaussian distribution, but frequently with right or left skew or differences in distribution according to sex.

This quantitative variability of morphometric traits is the basis for ethnic and family resemblance. Galtonian analysis is quintessentially the *quantitative* analysis of family resemblance. In clinical practice we may measure a few characteristics, such as head circumference, intercanthal distances, length of upper lip or length of ears; however, most of the time we enter subjective judgments and descriptions into the chart, frequently supplemented with photographic documentation.

Some of these traits are difficult to quantitate in clinical practice, the most prominent being ear position. Calling it "low-set ears" does not necessarily make it so, and on photos submitted to me, either for consultation or editorial evaluation, I frequently note that the ears do not appear to be low-set, but rather too large or too small, posteriorly angulated, and/or abnormally differentiated. There is, therefore, perhaps some merit to inserting almost always the word "apparently" in front of a clinical notation of low-set ears.

Individually, minor anomalies are indistinguishable from normal developmental variants. Minor anomalies are the commonest abnormality of development in aneuploidy syndromes where the multitude and greater or lesser severity of involvement leads to an abolishment of family resemblance.

In evaluating a given child or infant with apparent multiple minor anomalies, it is important to keep in mind the concept of the VFDP or "variant familial developmental pattern." In most FLK cases ("funny looking kid"—a term to be avoided) the child turns out to have a VFDP on examination of available first-degree relatives. Parents and grandparents are, as a matter of fact, extremely skillful in doing subjective analyses of family resemblance, and one of the most poignant indicators in infancy of the presence of an aneuploidy syndrome is their sad admission that the infant really does not look at all like anybody from either side of the family.

Thus, in determining whether a child has multiple minor anomalies or a VFDP it is important to do an analysis of family resemblance before deciding to inflict the pain and cost of a chromosome analysis on the child and family.

Before leaving the subject of minor anomalies it is important to reiterate the distinction between minor anomalies and mild malformations [23]. The latter are anomalies of organogenesis, and, regardless of how common in the population or how clinically innocuous, they are *always* abnormal all-or-none defects of morphogenetic thresholds. Minor anomalies are graded, mild malformations are present or absent; the former are almost by definition "polygenic" traits, the latter are more often mendelian (autosomal dominant) traits.

DEFORMITIES

The IWG [2] defined deformities as "abnormal form, shape, or position of a body part caused by mechanical forces." The pathogenetic analysis of deformities is relatively easy. In the craniofacial region these include plagiocephaly and plano-occiput commonly seen as secondary manifestation of congenital hypotonia. However, the skull deformity of the "breech baby" and of the premature infant is also well known. There are numerous craniosynostosis-associated changes of skull shape including the Kleeblattschädel or cloverleaf skull, and various combinations of acrocephaly, turribrachycephaly, dolichocephaly, etc, so nicely illustrated by Michael Cohen [24]. Deformities of auricles include anteversion and anteflexion, but also the flat auricles virtually devoid of secondary morphologic landmarks as seen in the Potter oligohydramnios sequence and in other cases where it can be presumed that intrinsic muscle function of the auricles was deficient. Flat philtrum, correlated with thin upper lip vermilion, must also be considered a deformity, probably together with the puckers and dimples seen on the chin in individuals with the Freeman-Sheldon syndrome.

By all odds the most common deformity sequences seen in the craniofacial region, also in many normal individuals, is that due to congenital hypotonia with prolonged persistence of flat bridge of nose, epicanthic folds, elongation of the upper lip, flattening of philtrum, anteversion of nostrils, inverted V-shaped configuration of the upper lip, mild micrognathia (which may disappear later on), high and narrowly arched palate, mild anterior neck webbing, etc. To some extent, similar anomalies may be present in cases of congenital weakness, which are much rarer and are exemplified by the weakness seen in congenital myotonic dystrophy.

SYNDROME

A syndrome, as used by geneticists, was redefined in causal terms at the 7th International Congress of Human Genetics in Berlin [3]. A syndrome in a genetic sense is now understood as a causally *homogeneous* complex of anomalies implying, at least in Mendelian traits, the concept of pleiotropy.

TABLE 1. The Acrofacial Dysostoses—Broadly Speaking

Reynolds–Webb syndrome
Nager syndrome
Genée–Wiedemann syndrome (or POADS) [26–28]
Fontaine syndrome
Kelly syndrome
Wyers syndrome
Townes–Brocks syndrome
Aneuploidy syndromes
duplication distal (2q),
trisomy 18, trisomy 21,
trisomy 7 mosaicism

However, it is probably not incorrect to extend the concept of pleiotropy, as least in genetic syndromes, also to aneuploidy syndromes.

In contradistinction, a field defect is, by definition, a causally *heterogeneous* complex of anomalies representing a disturbance of organogenesis, that is to say, of morphogenetic relationships including determination and induction.

Thus, the question arises, should it be Nager "syndrome" or "complex" (in the sense of a field defect)? This brings up the concept of the acrofacial dysostoses, which represent the combination of mandibulofacial dysostosis with pre- and/or postaxial acral (mostly hand) developmental defects. The fact that the combination of mandibulofacial dysostosis with radial ray abnormalities is causally heterogeneous, makes it, to my mind, more likely a polytopic developmental field defect, rather than a syndrome. Thus, the table of Reynolds et al [25] can be modified as shown in Table 1.

This correlation between mandibulofacial dysostosis and acral developmental field defects is as strong, if not stronger, than between kidney and limb anomalies in the acrorenal complex or polytopic field defect. It suggests that Janet McCredie may be right after all in that neural crest may have something to do with limb development [29].

Thus, there exists quite likely an acrofacial polytopic field defect, but also a causally unique Nager syndrome of the type first described by Nager and de Reynier [30].

EPISTEMOLOGY OF CRANIOFACIAL ANOMALIES

When accepting his invitation I promised the distinguished Chairman of this symposium not to stray too far into basic developmental biology; however, in this context I think it is important as a minimum to enumerate the cardinal epistemological characteristics of malformations in an attempt at further understanding of basic biology.

The three cardinal attributes of malformations are 1) presence/absence, which involves *causality;* 2) variability, which involves *pathogenesis;* 3) *phylogeneity,* which pertains to the evolution of field properties.

Presence/Absence

In this category phenomena can be ordered into four groups subdivided into two classes, namely those involving genetically normal and those involving gentically abnormal individuals.

Genetically normal. 1) In this category individuals may have normal development (the most common and most desirable state of affairs, but one that is highly uninformative), or b) abnormal development most commonly under teratogenic influence or as a consequence of abnormal maternal-fetal interaction as in maternal diabetes or maternal PKU.

In this connection, it is of interest to note that additional evidence is accumulating to support Thad Kelly's provocative hypothesis that some of the apparent components of the diphenylhydantoin syndrome appear to represent the inherited predisposition to epilepsy, rather than the direct developmental effect of dilantin [31–33].

Genetically abnormal. c) In those with normal development with respect to the trait, one speaks either of non-penetrance or, less commonly, of reduced phenotrance. d) In most cases those genetically abnormal for the trait will also be developmentally abnormal.

Variability

Qualitative variability affecting types and patterns of developmental defects. In Mendelian traits this involves the concept of *pleiotropy,* i.e., of one gene producing or being responsible for multiple different manifestations that may be produced at different times during development. In this connection it is important to note that the first pleiotropic gene affecting craniofacial and acral development, namely the autosomal dominant mutation responsible for the Greig syndrome, has been mapped successfully, in this case to 7p13 [34]. An oft quoted example of *mosaic pleiotropy* is the Ellis-van Creveld syndrome where the genetically correlated presence of polydactyly, skeletal dysplasia with dwarfism, congenital heart defects, and multiple buccal frenula cannot be readily correlated pathogenetically. An equally frequently cited example of *relational pleiotropy* is that of the connective tissue dysplasias, specifically the Marfan syndrome in which all of the ocular, cardiovascular, and musculoskeletal manifestations can be attributed to a pathogenetically and causally highly correlated intercellular disturbance of connective tissue function. However, occasionally pleiotropy encompasses a concept extending beyond the individual to several different relatives in a family. This was nicely illustrated by Toriello and Higgins [35] in their description of an X-linked mutation that produced in one individual stenosis of the aqueduct of Sylvius and hypospadias, in another anencephaly, in a third bilateral renal agenesis, in a fourth tetralogy of Fallot, and in a fifth cleft lip.

Quantitative variability is usually subsumed in a clinical context under the head of "severity" of the trait. Modifications of phenotype may be *epistatic* in the narrow sense defined by Bateson [36] of suppression of the function of a gene or allele through action of a gene or allele at a different locus or *epigenetic* in the broader sense defined by Waddington [37], namely of the influence of many genes interacting with the environment on the expression of the phenotype.

Phylogeneity

It was necessary to coin this term to describe the phenomenon well-documented by many investigators in the 19th century of the occurrence of the apparently identical malformation, such as otocephaly or cyclopia, in different, more or less closely related species. Some of these malformations are *atavistic,* as in the ontogenetic restoration of the ancestral pentadactylous foot in the guinea pig or in horses with 3 or 5 fully developed toes. However, most are non-atavistic malformations, such as true polydactyly of the horse or the cyclopia that has been seen or produced in dozens of teleostean, avian, and mammalian species.

Phylogeneity implies an identical manner of disturbance of morphogenesis in fields identical in the several species under discussion because of descent from an ancestor with a prototypic developmental plan.

Phylogeneity has several important implications for understanding normal and abnormal human development.

The first is that genes involved in evolutionary changes are probably also involved in normal ontogeny.

Second, specific malformations seen in two or more non-human species are also ultimately to be expected in humans.

Third, what appears to have been conserved in evolution is the extraordinary economy, uniformity, stability, and conservatism of developmental paths, rather than the details of the genetic messages coding for the paths, in accord with the message on the bumper sticker of our Hospital Administrator and in the latest manuscript by Murphy et al on "Angular Homeostasis" [38], namely "if it works, don't fix it!"

In a homely manner this concept can be illustrated by restating the clock metaphor in a different manner. Clocks can evidently be made of plastic, metal, wood, and sometimes even of paper, they can be large or small, they come in different colors and models, prominently visible in public buildings, sitting on desks, carried around wrists, or put in pockets on the end of a chain. None of these variations matter so long as the big hand goes around the dial once an hour, and the small one once every 24 hours. Furthermore, the instructions can be given not only in the several languages written in the Latin alphabet, but also those written in the Greek, Cyrillic, Arabic, Chinese, and many other alphabets.

All of this is to confirm once more what Sewall Wright said all of his life, namely that recapitulation and the focus of Darwinian selection involves primarily phenotypes and only secondarily genotypes.

ACKNOWLEDGMENTS

I am deeply grateful for the expert secretarial collaboration of Mrs. Marilyn Nicolay.

REFERENCES

1. His W: "Die Anatomische Nomenclatur. Nomina Anatomica." Verzeichniss der von der Anatomischen Gesellschaft auf ihrer IX. Versammlung in Basel angenommenen Namen. Leipzig: Verlag von Veit and Co., 1895.
2. Spranger J, Benirschke K, Hall JG, Lenz W, Lowry RB, Opitz JM, Pinsky L, Schwarzacher JG, Smith DW: Errors of morphogenesis, concepts and terms. Recommendations of an International Working Group. J Pediatr 100:160–165, 1982.
3. Opitz JM, Czeizel A, Evans JA, Hall JG, Lubinsky MS, Spranger JW: Nosologic groupings in birth defects. In: Vogel F, Sperling K (eds): "Human Genetics." Heidelberg: Springer Verlag, 1987.
4. Galton F: "Natural Inheritance." New York: MacMillan and Co., 1889.
5. LeDouarin N: "The Neural Crest." New York: Cambridge University Press, 1982.
6. Noden DM: Origins and patterning of craniofacial mesenchymal tissues. J Craniofac Genet Dev Biol 6 (Suppl 2):15–31, 1986.
7. Opitz JM: The developmental field concept. Am J Med Genet 21:1–11, 1985.
8. Opitz JM: Editorial Comment: Developmental field theory and observations—Accidental progress? Am J Med Genet 25 (Suppl 2):1–8, 1986.
9. Bolande RP: The neurocristopathies. A unifying concept of disease arising in neural crest maldevelopment. Hum Pathol 5:409–429, 1974.
10. Johnston MC: The neural crest in abnormalities of the face and brain. Birth Defects XI(7):1–18, 1975.
11. Kaplan P, de Chadarévian J-P: Piebaldism-Waardenburg syndrome: Histopathologic evidence for a neurocristopathy. Am J Med Genet 31:679–688, 1988.
12. Gluecksohn-Waelsch S: [re oel mouse]. Mouse Newslett 25:12ff, 1960.
13. Spiegelman M, Bennett D: Fine structural study of cell migration in early mesoderm of normal and mutant mouse embryo (T-locus t^9/t^9). J Embryol Exp Morphol 32:723–738, 1974.
14. Waterman RE: Scanning electron microscope studies of central nervous system development. Birth Defects XV(3):55–77, 1979.

15. Morriss GM: Morphogenesis of the malformations induced in rat embryos by maternal hypervitaminosis A. J Anat 133:241–250, 1972.
16. Hassell J, Greenberg JA, Johnston MC: Inhibition of cranial neural crest cell development by vitamin A in the chick embryo. J Embryol Exp Morphol 39:267, 1977.
17. Lammer EJ, Opitz JM: The DiGeorge anomaly as a developmental field defect. Am J Med Genet 25 (Suppl 2):113–127, 1986.
18. Johnston MC, Sulik KK: Some abnormal patterns of development in the craniofacial region. Birth Defects XV(8):23–42, 1979.
19. Holthusen W, Birtel T, Brinkmann H, Gunkel J, Janneck C, Richter E: Die Currarino-Triade. Fortschr Röntgenstr 143:83–89, 1988.
20. Penchaszadeh VB, Velasques D, Arrivillaga R: The nasopalpebral lipoma-coloboma syndrome: A new autosomal dominant dysplasia-malformation syndrome with congenital nasopalpebral lipomas, eyelid colobomas, telecanthus, and maxillary hypoplasia. Am J Med Genet 11:397–410, 1982.
21. Bonner-Fraser M: Perturbation of cranial neural crest migration by the HNK-1 antibody. Dev Biol 123:321–331, 1987.
22. Abbott NJ: The milieu is the message. Nature 332:490,491, 1988.
23. Opitz JM: Invited Editorial Comment: Study of minor anomalies in childhood malignancy. Eur J Pediatr 144:252–254, 1985.
24. Cohen MM, Jr: Craniosynostosis update. Am J Med Genet 30 (Suppl 4):99–148, 1988.
25. Reynolds JF, Webb MJ, Opitz JM: A new autosomal dominant acrofacial dysostosis syndrome. Am J Med Genet 25 (Suppl 2):143–150, 1986.
26. Opitz JM: Editorial Comment: Nager ''syndrome'' versus ''anomaly'' and its nosology with the postaxial acrofacial dysostosis syndrome of Genée and Wiedemann. Am J Med Genet 27:959–963, 1987.
27. Meinecke P, Wiedemann H-R: Robin sequence and oligodactyly in mother and son—Probably a further example of the postaxial acrofacial dysostosis syndrome. (Letter) Am J Med Genet 27:953–956, 1987.
28. Opitz JM, Stickler GB: The Genée-Wiedemann syndrome, an acrofacial dysostosis—Further observation. (Letter) Am J Med Genet 27:971–975, 1987.
29. McCredie J: Neural crest defects. A neuroanatomic basis for classification of multiple malformations related to phocomelia. J Neurol Sci 28:373–387, 1976.
30. Nager FR, de Reynier JP: Das Gehörorgan bei den angeborenen Kopfmissbildungen. Pract Oto-Rhino-Laryngol (Basel) 10(Suppl 2):1–128, 1948.
31. Kelly TE, Edwards P, Rein M, Miller JQ, Dreifuss FE: Teratogenicity of anticonvulsant drugs. II: A prospective study. Am J Med Genet 19:435–443, 1984.
32. Gaily E, Granstrom M-L, Hiilesmaa V, Bardy A: Minor anomalies in offspring of epileptic mothers. J Pediatr 112:520–529, 1988.
33. Holmes LB: Teratogenic effects of anticonvulsant drugs. J Pediatr 112:579–581, 1988.
34. Brueton L, Huson SM, Winter RM, Williamson R: The chromosomal localization of a developmental gene in man: Direct DNA analysis demonstrates that Greig cephalopolysyndactyly (GCPS) maps to 7p13. Am J Med Genet 31:799–804, 1988.
35. Toriello HV, Higgins JV: X-linked midline defects. Am J Med Genet 21:143–146, 1985.
36. Bateson W: The progress of genetics since the rediscovery of Mendel's paper. Prog Rei Bot 1:368, 1907.
37. Waddington CH: The genetic control of wing development in *Drosophila*. J Genet 41:75, 1985.
38. Murphy EA, Berger KR, Trojak JE, Sagawa Y: Angular homeostasis 5. Some issues in genetics, ontogeny and evolution. Am J Med Genet 31:963–979, 1988.

Craniofacial Manifestations of Ehlers-Danlos Syndromes, Cutis Laxa Syndromes, and Cutis Laxa-Like Syndromes

Robert J. Gorlin, DDS, MS, and Michael M. Cohen, Jr., DMD, PhD

Department of Oral Pathology & Genetics, University of Minnesota School of Dentistry, Minneapolis, MN 55455 (R.J.G.), and Department of Oral Pathology, Faculty of Dentistry, Dalhousie University, Halifax, Nova Scotia, Canada (M.M.C.)

Although our original assignment was to cover the oral manifestations of all connective tissue diseases, osteogenesis imperfecta and Marfan syndrome are being superbly covered in other sections of these proceedings. Therefore, we will limit ourselves to a discussion of the Ehlers-Danlos syndromes, the cutis laxa syndromes, gerodermia osteodysplastica, De Barsy syndrome, and Wiedemann-Rautenstrauch syndrome.

DE BARSY SYNDROME

De Barsy et al [1] and others [2–8] described a syndrome of intrauterine growth retardation, wrinkled atrophic skin, open fontanels and sutures, somatic and mental retardation, brisk deep tendon reflexes, athetoid posturing, hypermobility of small joints, and muscular hypotonia. The facies is characterized by frontal bossing in early childhood, but postnatal changes include microcephaly, prematurely aged appearance, corneal clouding, large dysplastic ears, hypertelorism, and thin lips (Fig. 1). Some patients have cataracts. We are not convinced that the child noted by Bartsocas [9] has the syndrome. Inheritance may be autosomal recessive [7].

Elastic fibers are frayed and reduced in number. Chemotactic migration of cultured fibroblasts is reduced, and there is impaired granulocyte function [4,6]. The disorder must be differentiated from *cutis laxa syndromes* and those of premature aging (acrogeria, metagyria, and *gerodermia osteodysplastica*).

GERODERMIA OSTEODYPLASTICA (BAMATTER SYNDROME)

The family first reported by Bamatter et al [10], in 1949, was reviewed by the same group of investigators over a 20-year period [11–13]. The disorder

Birth Defects: Original Article Series, Volume 25, Number 4, pages 39–71

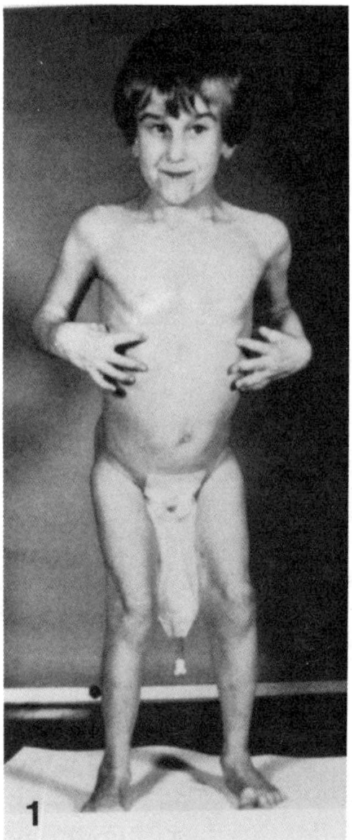

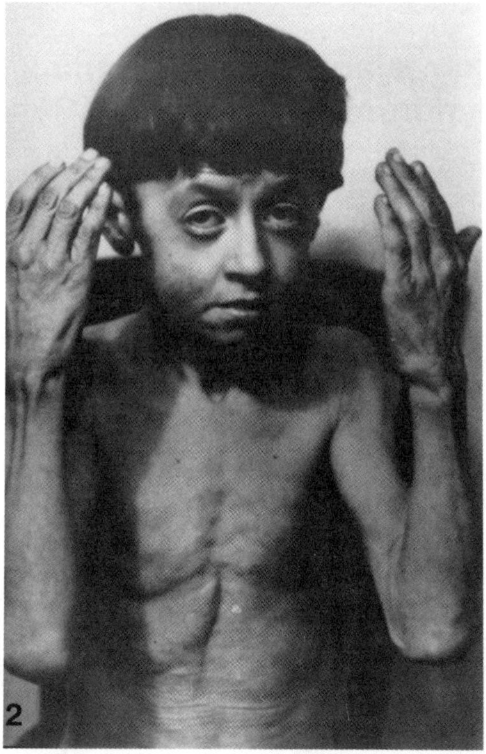

Fig. 1. *De Barsy syndrome*. Athetoid posturing, wrinkled atrophic skin, sagging cheeks, and contractures at knees. Child is mentally retarded.

Fig. 2. *Gerodermia osteodysplastica*. Because of looseness of facial skin, there is a sad appearance. The eyelids and cheeks droop. The skin is thin and without turgor over the hands (from G. Boreaux [12]).

has a characteristic facies, hyperlaxity of skin and joints, and growth retardation (Fig. 2). Other families have been reported. In the interest of linguistic purity [14,15], we have changed the name from geroderma osteodysplastia to gerodermia osteodysplastica [16].

Originally thought to be X-linked [13], recent evidence suggests autosomal recessive inheritance [14,17].

Growth retardation is below the third percentile in perhaps one-third of the children. Frequently, span is greater than height.

Facies

Owing to looseness of the skin, a sad appearance is imparted. The eyelids and cheeks droop. The head tends to be brachycephalic. The forehead is prominent. The nose is often jutting and fleshy. The lower lip is downturned, and the midface is frequently mildly hypoplastic with relative mandibular prognathism. About one-half of the patients exhibit malar flush.

Skin

The skin is thin and creased with recoil. It is especially without turgor over the hands and feet.

Musculoskeletal

Constant features are marked muscular hypotonia and hyperlaxity of joints (hands, feet, knees, hips) with associated hernias, flat feet, and dislocated hips. Inguinal hernia has been found in approximately 35%. A virtually constant feature is osteoporosis with resultant platyspondyly, anterior wedging, and occasionally biconcave vertebral bodies [18]. Compression fractures may be observed within the first few years of life. Long bones tend to fracture with minimal trauma. Mild scoliosis and sternal anomalies are present in about 65%. Radiographic changes include multiple wormian bones in lambdoidal suture.

Oral Manifestation

At least 70% have downturned lower lip. Almost constant features are malocclusion and highly arched palate. The alveolar bone is decreased in amount.

Differential Diagnosis

Gerodermia osteodysplastica is most likely to be confused with the *cutis laxa syndromes*. Acrogeria is characterized by wrinkled and aged-appearing skin, most marked over the dorsa of the hands and feet, flat feet, and dislocated hips. However, in gerodermia osteodysplastica, the skin is not atrophic, and the superficial veins are not highly visible. Commonly associated with acrogeria are wide cranial sutures, blue sclerae, diaphyseal narrowing of long bones, and nail dysplasia. Furthermore, individuals who have acrogeria are not jowly nor do they exhibit the joint hyperextensibility and the osteoporotic bony changes seen here.

The syndrome should be differentiated from wrinkly skin syndrome reported by Gazit et al [19]. This autosomal recessively inherited disorder is characterized by wrinkled skin of the anterior chest and/or dorsal surfaces of the hands, hypotonia, kyphosis, winged scapulas, and prominent cutaneous venous pattern. There are also microcephaly, severe myopia, and chorioretinitis.

The *De Barsy syndrome,* characterized by congenital atheotosis, mental retardation, severe growth retardation, and laxity of skin and ligaments, must also be excluded.

Lenz-Majewski syndrome and *Patterson syndrome* (pseudo-leprechaunism) have wrinkly skin as one of their components, but the phenotypes of those disorders are so distinct that discussion is not relevant.

CUTIS LAXA SYNDROMES

Cutis laxa is characterized by skin that hangs in loose folds. There are many forms, some genetic, others acquired. Confusion existed in the early literature since the Ehlers-Danlos syndromes (EDS) also had that designation. While the term *cutis laxa* was used as early as 1833 by Alibert [20], the generalized form was probably first described by Graf [21] in 1836. A good general review is that of Mensing et al [22].

Autosomal Recessive Form

This is the most common congenital genetic type of cutis laxa. Birthweight is normal, but often there is mild postnatal growth deficiency. Most of these children die by the 3rd year of life.

Affected sibs [23–26] and parental consanguinity [25,27–31] indicate autosomal recessive inheritance. We believe that the syndrome reported by Dallaire et al [32] does not represent a separate disorder as they suggest.

Facies and skin. Owing to accentuation of skin folds, the infant appears aged (Fig. 3). The upper lip is long and the columella is short. Blepharochalasis and, at times, ectropion add to the aged appearance [22,33,34]. The skin of the entire body appears too large. There is no hyperelasticity, fragility, or difficulty in healing.

Cardiorespiratory. Tachypnea, pneumonitis, and airway obstruction associated with emphysema are common features. This results in severe hypoxemia, respiratory failure, cor pulmonale, and right ventricular enlargement. These findings together with diaphragmatic hernia lead to early demise [23,26,33,34]. The emphysema results from generalized elastolysis. Bundle branch block [23], pulmonary artery stenosis [24,31], and dilated and tortuous carotid, vertebral, and pulmonary arteries and aortic root [23,31,35] have been noted.

Musculoskeletal. Hernia is common: inguinal [23,24,26,27,34,36], diaphragmatic [23,27,30.37], ventral, and/or umbilical [23,26]. Loose joints are rarely noted [27].

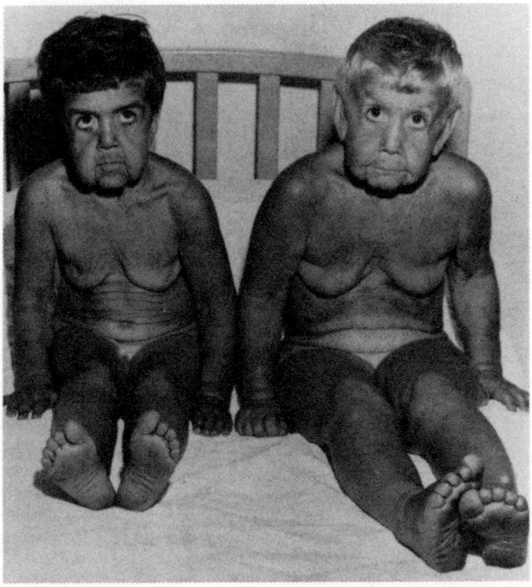

Fig. 3. *Cutis laxa*. Affected sibs with autosomal recessive type of cutis laxa look much older than their chronologic ages of 5 and 6 years. (Courtesy of F.A. Balboni, Garden City, New York.)

Gastrointestinal. Diverticula of the gastrointestinal tract have been documented: pharynx [29], esophagus [23,34], and rectum [23–26].

Genitourinary. Bladder diverticula have been described by several authors [23,26,27,29,38,39]. Vaginal prolapse has also been noted.

Oral. The voice is deep and resonant in quality because of a laxity of the vocal cords [23,39,40]. There is also looseness of the oral and pharyngeal mucosa [23].

Autosomal Dominant Form

This form is less common than the autosomal recessive type and runs a quite benign course [30,34,35,39,41–47]. Perhaps the earliest published example is that of Rossbach [48] in 1884. Onset is usually somewhat later than the recessive form. Drooping of eyelids and sagging facial skin together with accentuation of the nasolabial and other facial folds produce an aged appearance. The nose is often hooked, the nostrils are everted, and the philtrum is long. An affected pubertal child will often look older than the unaffected parent! Complications are few, and lifespan is normal.

Rarely associated abnormalities have included hoarseness [41–43], pulmonary artery stenosis [35,43], mitral valve prolapse [42], hernia [30], bronchiectasis [39], joint dislocations [42], tortuosity and dilatation of carotid arteries and aorta [43,49], dilatation of sinuses of Valsalva [42], and coarctation of aorta [41].

Cutis Laxa, Late Closure of Fontanels, Intrauterine Growth Retardation, and Hyperlaxity of Joints

Debré et al [50], in 1937, were possibly the first to describe this form of cutis laxa. Several other authors have reported examples [27,51–65]. It should be noted that the patient reported by Theopold and Wildhack [65] is a cousin of the patients reported by Fittke [53]. Possibly the patient described by Schirren et al [66] had this condition. Inheritance is probably autosomal recessive, but most patients are female [57,60,63,64]. The rate of parental consanguinity is high.

Birthweight and length are under the 10th percentile. Delayed postnatal growth, mild gross motor retardation, poor feeding, and mild mental retardation have been common. Sagging jowls, epicanthic folds, sunken nasal bridge, and apparent mild hypertelorism are common. In addition to congenital cutis laxa, which is especially severe over the abdomen, hands, and feet, there is late closure of the fontanels, especially the anterior one. The skull sutures are markedly separated. The hips, either one or more, often both, are congenitally dislocated in 85%. All joints exhibit generalized laxity, especially those of the hands, which leads to unusual positioning. All appear to have fifth finger clinodactyly. Talipes equinovarus has been noted in a few cases. The subcutaneous veins of the abdomen are markedly dilated, and the abdominal musculature is lax. Inguinal hernia has been found. Less constant findings include downslanting palpebral fissures, macular coloboma, myopia, iris hypoplasia, single transverse palmar crease, and hydronephrosis [51,66]. Cleft lip has been reported [60].

Differential diagnosis. X-linked cutis laxa is now called *Ehlers-Danlos syndrome, type IX.*

Acquired cutis laxa may follow nonspecific cutaneous inflammation or persistent urticaria. Occasionally there is no history of prior skin disorder. Some patients have only cutaneous involvement, while others have internal manifestations: pulmonary emphysema with cardiovascular complications, femoral, inguinal, ventral, or diaphragmatic hernias, diverticula of the intestinal tract, cystocele, rectocele, and uterine prolapse [29,67–69]. Ruptured patellar tendons and associated multiple myeloma have been reported

[70,71]. The reader is referred to several thorough reviews of acquired cutis laxa [40,72–75].

Braun-Falco et al [76] were dealing with a case of prune belly. Tracheobronchiomegaly (Mounier-Kuhn syndrome) is characterized by dilatation and diverticulas of the trachea and bronchi [77] with blepharochalasis and redundancy of oral mucosa *(Ascher syndrome).* The "wrinkly" skin syndrome, a recessively inherited disorder, characterized by congenital wrinkling of the skin of the chest, abdomen, and dorsa of the hands and feet, must be excluded. The palms and soles have increased numbers of wrinkles. There is generalized hypotonia with winging of the scapulae [19].

Cutis laxa has also been found in association with a dominantly inherited syndrome of corneal lattice dystrophy, cranial nerve palsy and nephropathy [78]. It has also been seen with severe osteoporosis [79]. *Gerodermia osteodysplastica, De Barsy syndrome,* and *Lenz-Majewski syndrome* should be excluded. Each is associated with cutis laxa. A congenital generalized cutis laxa may result from chronic maternal penicillamine therapy during pregnancy. These infants may have severe pulmonary complications [75,80,81].

Bladder diverticula may also be seen in Menkes syndrome, prune belly sequence, *Ehlers-Danlos syndromes,* and *Williams syndrome.*

Pathology. With orcein or Weigert elastic fiber stain, absence or marked diminution of elastic fibers has been observed especially in the papillary layer of the dermis. Degenerative changes are marked by fragmentation of elastic fibers. Some fibers are short and thin.

Ultrastructural changes include normal microfibril formation, deficiency of elastin, and uneven distribution of dense amorphous or granular substances that produce dense bundles [82–85]. The various types of cutis laxa cannot be differentiated by light or electron microscopic study.

Laboratory aids. The mechanism by which there is insufficient elastin is not known. Whether it is based on deficient formation or accelerated destruction has not been shown. While low serum copper and increased elastase and/or decreased anti-elastase levels [23,33,82,86] have been reported, others have found normal or even elevated values [43,82]. Acquired cutis laxa is associated with normal enzyme levels [43].

WIEDEMANN-RAUTENSTRAUCH SYNDROME

In 1977, Rautenstrauch et al [87], believing that they were dealing with progeria in sibs, described a new progeroid syndrome, which was recognized as such by Wiedemann [88]. An aged facies is present from birth (Figure 4). Children are born small for dates, and subsequent growth is slow. Frontal and biparietal bossing, together with small facial bones, gives the child a hydrocephalic appearance. The anterior fontanel is large and closes late. The

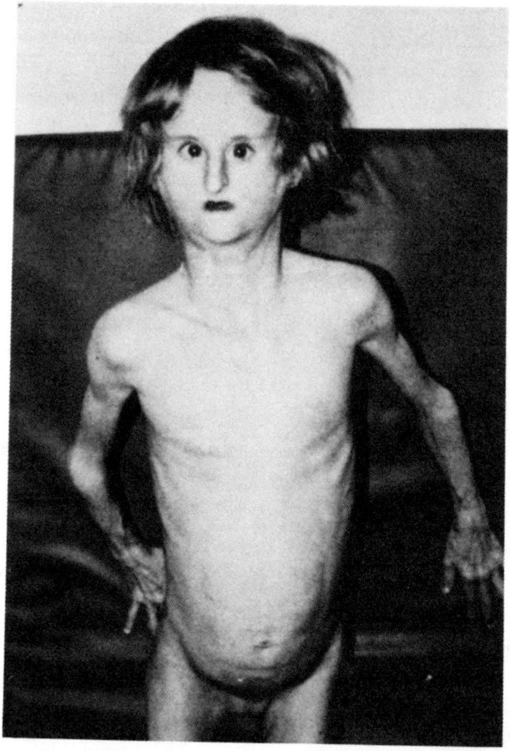

Fig. 4. *Wiedemann-Rautenstrauch syndrome*. Small facial bones give patient appearance of hydrocephalus. Note small beaked nose and microstomia (from T. Rautenstrauch et al [87]).

sutures tend to persist. Scalp hair tends to be sparse but is of normal consistency. The scalp veins are prominent. The nose is small and beaked, and the ears are low-set and posteriorly angulated. The facial bones are hypoplastic. The mouth is small, and the chin is somewhat prominent [89,90]. Natal incisors are consistently present [89].

Subcutaneous fat is generally reduced, allowing the veins and muscles to become prominent, but caudal fat accumulates during infancy. The abdomen is prominent. The hands and feet are large with long fingers and toes.

Mental and, especially, motor development are usually deficient. Horizontal nystagmus is noted with limited visual acuity [85]. There is progressive neurologic degeneration by the age of 5 years. Lack of head control, hypotonia, severe truncal ataxia, dysmetria, and intension tremor are common. Martin et al [91] found extensive demyelinization of the central nervous system with occasional tigroid pattern and large amounts of neutral fat and myelin breakdown in macrophages, a picture characteristic of pure sudanophilic leukodystrophy. Recurrent respiratory tract infections are common. Most of the children die prior to the age of 5 years.

Inheritance is clearly autosomal recessive [87,92]. To date, study of collagen has not been fruitful [89].

EHLERS-DANLOS SYNDROME

Introduction

The Ehlers-Danlos syndromes constitute a heterogeneous group of generalized connective tissue disorders with skin fragility, skin hyperextensibility, and joint hypermobility (Table 1). The earliest recognized description was of a young Spaniard, George Albes, who was exhibited to the Academy of Leyden in Holland in 1657 by van Meekeren [93,94]. The first scientific description was by Tschernogobow, a Russian dermatologist who presented an affected 17-year-old boy to the Moscow Venereology and Dermatology Society meeting in 1892. He attributed the multi-system features to a generalized defect in embryonic formation of connective tissue. Throughout the Soviet medical literature, the condition is known as Chernogubov syndrome [95].

Ehlers [96], in 1901, reported the association of hyperelastic skin, skin hemorrhages, and loose-jointedness. Danlos [97], in 1908, added cutaneous pseudotumors and fragility, and Weber and Aitken [98] added subcutaneous spherules. Terminology became especially complex during the early part of the 20th century. Among descriptive features used to name the condition were dermatorrhexis, dermatolysis, Gummihaut, cutis pendula, cutis hyperelastica, and chalasoderma. The eponym Ehlers-Danlos syndrome finally emerged as the name used most commonly in the West.

More than 500 affected individuals had been reported in over 300 articles by 1982. Comprehensive surveys are those of McKusick [94], Beighton et al [93,99,100], and Hollister et al [101,102]. The reader is referred to the following references for detailed coverage: molecular defects and connective tissue metabolism [103–108]; ultrastructural studies of the skin [109–111]; histologic studies of the skin [112]; collagen studies [113–115]; cardiovascular abnormalities [116–117]; and pregnancy [118].

During the last several years, genetic and biochemical studies have defined more than ten types of Ehlers-Danlos syndrome, and the molecular basis of several of them has been identified. It is important to specify the type of Ehlers-Danlos syndrome a patient has because the natural history and mode of inheritance differ, depending upon type. Clinical features, inheritance, and the biochemical defect of various forms are summarized in Table

TABLE 1. Clinical Features, Modes of Inheritance, and Biochemical Defects in Ehlers-Danlos Syndromes

Type	Clinical features	Inheritance	Biochemical defect
I: Gravis	Soft velvety, hyperextensible skin; easy bruising; "cigarette paper" scars; hypermobile joints; varicose veins; prematurity	AD	Not known
II: Mitis	Similar to Ehlers-Danlos type I, but less severe	AD	Not known
III: Familial hypermobility	Soft skin, no scarring, marked large and small joint hypermobility	AD	Not known
IV: Arterial	Thin, translucent skin with visible veins; marked bruising; skin and joints have normal extensibility; arterial, bowel, and uterine rupture	AD,AR	Abnormal type III, collagen synthesis, secretion, or structure
V: X-linked	Similar to Ehlers-Danlos type II	SLR	Not known
VI: Ocular	Soft, velvety, hyperextensible skin; hypermobile joints; scoliosis; ocular fragility and keratoconus	AR	Lysyl hydroxylase deficiency
VII: Arthrochalasis multiplex congenita	Congenital hip dislocation; joint hypermobility; soft skin with normal scarring	AD	Structural mutation at amino-terminal cleavage site in pro 1 (I) and pro 2 (I) defective aminopeptidase
VIII: Periodontal*	Generalized periodontitis; skin similar to Ehlers-Danlos type II	AD	Not known
IX: Cutis laxa, bladder diverticulae, occipital horns**	Soft extensible, lax skin; bladder diverticulae and rupture; short arms; limited pronation and supination; broad clavicles; occipital horns	XLR	Abnormal copper utilization with defect in lysyl oxidase
X: Fibronectin	Similar to Ehlers-Danlos type II	AR	Defect in fibronectin

*Probably same as type IV.

**Sometimes classified as form of cutis laxa.

1. Besides types I–X, several other types are listed by name but are not numbered as types. Approximately 80% of affected individuals have type I or type II. Approximately 10% have type III, about 4% have type IV, and about 6% have various other types [100].

Many patients with Ehlers-Danlos-like clinical findings do not fit the general classification, and as more biochemical studies are completed, it is likely that the classification will expand. From the clinical perspective, important considerations are the mode of inheritance and whether the natural history can be predicted from family or biochemical studies. It is vital to distinguish the recessively inherited form of type VI because prenatal diagnosis is potentially available. It is also important to identify patients with type IV so that clear discussion of pregnancy risks and problems of surgery can take place in a nonemergent setting. The initial evaluation of each patient should include careful physical examination and detailed family history. Biochemical studies of collagens synthesized by fibroblasts cultured from dermal punch biopsies can identify patients with type IV, type VI, and some patients with type VII. Low serum copper and ceruloplasmin levels identify patients with type IX. Defects in collagen processing or of the structure or synthesis of other matrix macromolecules will probably be identified in patients with types I and II in the future, and research in these areas is underway. Several laboratories in the United States, Great Britain, Europe, and Australia can provide the laboratory investigations needed to characterize the various types of Ehlers-Danlos syndrome.

Types I (Severe Form) and II (Mild Form)

Types I (severe form) and II (mild form) have autosomal dominant inheritance. Only rarely are they characterized by major complications. The clinical findings in both types may be dramatic with markedly soft, velvety hyperextensible skin, impressive joint hypermobility, easy bruising, and thin, atrophic, "cigarette-paper" scars (Fig. 5a–g). Varicose veins are common. Birth prevalence of these two disorders is estimated to be approximately 1/10–20,000 [93,94].

The biochemical bases of types I and II are not known. Early studies suggested that the solubility of dermal collagens was increased [119] and that skin tensile strength, contributed largely by collagen, was decreased [93]. More recently, morphologic studies have shown that the architecture of collagen fibrils in skin is unusual. Collagen fibril diameter is larger than normal, and there are multiple composite fibrils [107,115]. Shinkai et al [108] suggested that the cellular processing of type I collagen was not normal. The studies of P.H. Byers (personal communication, 1987) suggest that cleavage of the COOH-terminal propeptide extensions may be far slower than normal in cell culture. These findings are compatible with the sugges-

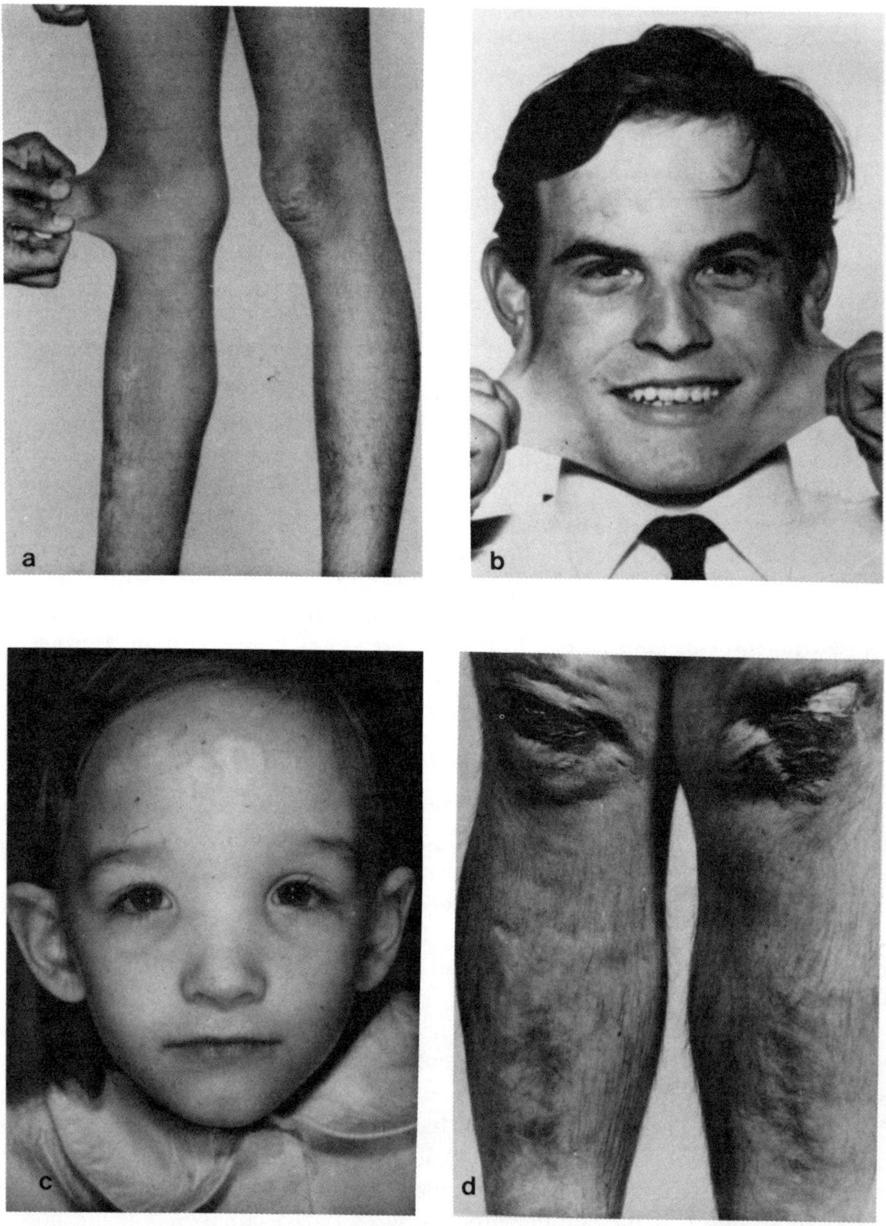

Fig. 5. *Ehlers-Danlos syndrome type I.* **a:** Extensive stretchability of skin. **b:** Hyperelastic skin returns to normal position after being stretched (from P.E. Beighton, "The Ehlers-Danlos Syndrome." London: Heinemann Med. Books, Ltd., 1970) [93]. **c:** Numerous "cigarette paper" scars of face, epicanthal folds, flat nasal bridge (from G.M. Barabas and A.P. Barabas [137]). **d:** Papyraceous scars of knees and atrophic scars of shins. **e:** Extreme joint hypermobility. **f:** Ability to touch nose with tongue tip, present in 50% of patients with Ehlers-Danlos syndrome, occurs in less than 10% of normal persons. **g:** Easy eversion of upper lids (Méténier sign) (from P.E. Beighton [93]).

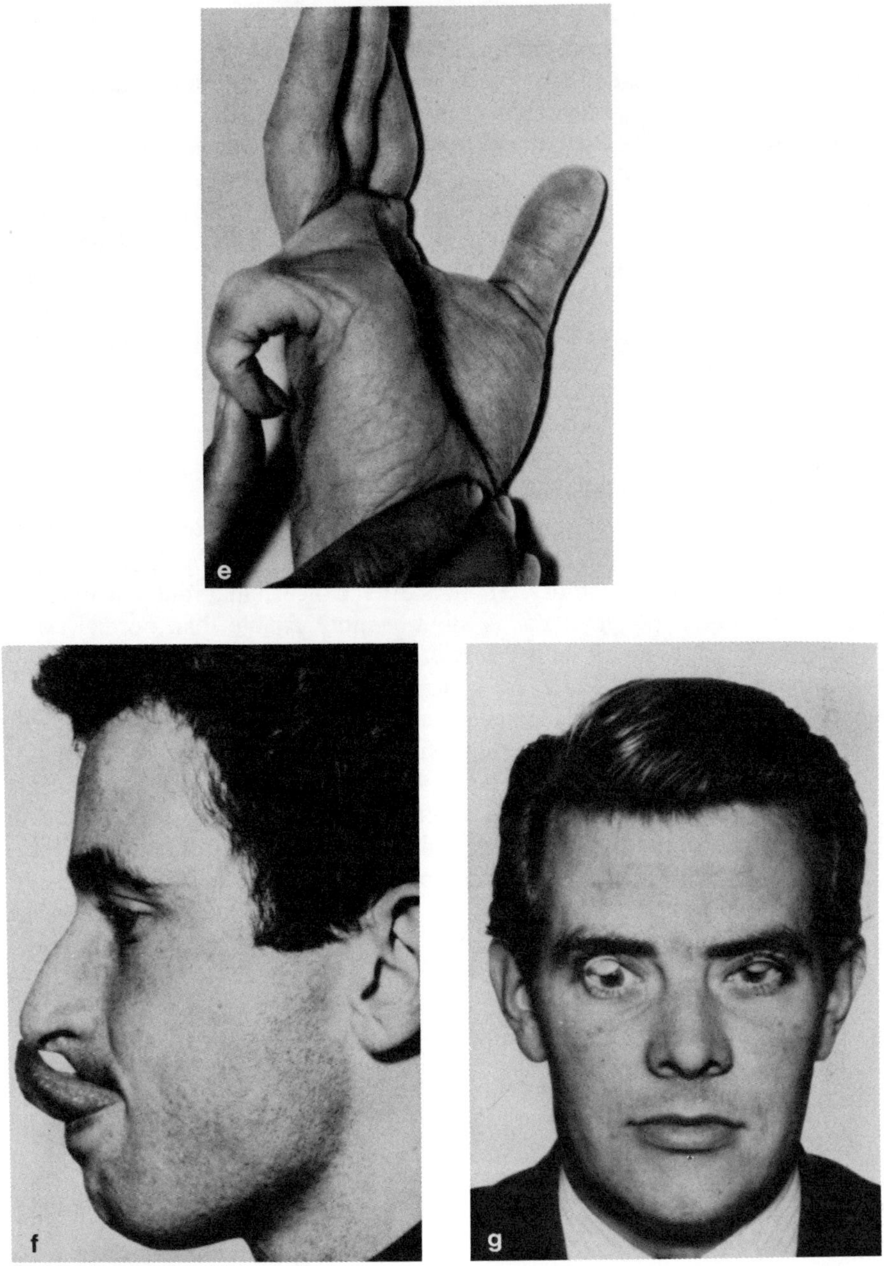
e
f
g

tions that type I procollagen, which retains COOH-terminal propeptide extensions, is unable to form normal fibril structures [113]. To date, linkage studies have not located the genes for type I and II. A family with reduced amounts of type III collagen has been documented [120].

General features. Prematurity, because of early rupture of fetal membranes, is observed in as many as one-half of type I cases [118,121–123] and to a lesser degree in type II cases. In addition, there may be postpartum hemorrhage, hemorrhage following episiotomy or lacerations, and uterine or bladder prolapse [123]. Children with type I or type II EDS are often thought to have joint hypermobility as newborns, but they may not come to medical attention until about 1 year when they are noted to be slow to walk because of poor joint stability. Susceptibility to skin tearing, forming of thin scars, and easy bruising becomes apparent. Evaluation for child abuse is not uncommon and should be guarded against [124]. Evidence of mitral valve prolapse by clinical criteria or by echocardiography may be present in childhood and certainly by adolescence.

Early onset of joint symptoms occurs, apparently resulting in premature osteoarthritis from mechanical stress on joints produced by excessive mobility and mild joint instability. There is often concern that routine surgery is hazardous, but although tissue is slightly more friable than normal, with careful attention to detail during surgical procedures, the likelihood of complication is minimal. Sutures are generally left in place two to three times longer than usual to assure adequate healing. Life expectancy for individuals with type I or type II Ehlers-Danlos syndromes is normal [92,94,101,102].

Skin. The skin has a velvety feel and is hyperelastic, especially over the major joints. After being stretched, it returns to its normal position. The skin is thinner than normal [125], brittle, and fragile. Minimal trauma may produce gaping wounds. After healing, pigmented papyraceous scars result. These can usually be detected over the forehead, chin, knees, shins, and/or elbows. Bruising is variable in degree. Goodman et al [126] demonstrated secondary skin creases over the palms.

Molluscoid pseudotumors over the heels and major joints are not uncommon, and often the skin is redundant on the hands and feet [127,128]. Calcified, cyst-like structures 2 to 10 mm in diameter may be found subcutaneously, especially over bony prominences of the forearms and shins in about 30% [129]. Varicose veins are common, and acrocyanosis has been noted with increased frequency.

Musculoskeletal system. Hyperextensibility of joints, weak hand clasp, and pes planus are usually present [130,131]. Genu recurvatum has been noted in about 25%, and there may be recurrent joint dislocations. Talipes has been found in approximately 5%. The ulnar styloid process may be elongated. Kyphoscoliosis and thoracic asymmetry are observed in 15–20%

but usually are not severe [129,131]. Hernia, either inguinal or umbilical, has been found in 10–20% [132].

Cardiovascular defects. Leier et al [117] studied 16 patients with type I. Roentgenograms, electrocardiograms, and echocardiograms were done. Many underwent cardiac catheterization. Most patients had mitral valve prolapse, and six had tricuspid valve prolapse. Dilatation of the aortic root or ectasia of the sinuses of Valsalva, or both, also occurred in six patients. Congenital heart defects included two cases of bicuspid aortic valve, one instance of pulmonic valvular stenosis, two VSDs, and one ASD.

Craniofacial features. Epicanthic folds are seen in about 25% [94, 127,128,133]. Blue sclerae are noted in less than 10% [127,128,131,134]. Myopia and strabismus have been observed with far greater frequency than blue sclerae. Also noted have been microcornea, retinal detachment, keratoconus, and angioid streaks [135,136]. Hyperextensibility of skin allows for easy eversion of the upper eyelids (Méténier's sign) [93]. The pinnae may project outward [134].

Approximately 50% can touch the nose with the tip of the tongue (Gorlin's sign), an ability found in only 8–10% of the general population. The oral mucosa is fragile and easily bruised. Oral healing may be slightly retarded, since the edges of a wound draw apart, but there is not evidence of abnormal healing or excessive scar formation in the mouth [137]. The gingiva are more liable to injury, and periodontal disease may occur at an earlier age [127,128]. Recurrent subluxation of the temporomandibular joint has been reported [130,138,139].

Barabas and Barabas [137] found that premolar and molar teeth had high cusps and deep occlusal fissures. Roentgenographically, teeth may have stunted and deformed roots and large pulp stones in the coronal part of the pulp chamber [137,140–144]. Barabas [140] found hypoplastic areas in enamel, irregularities of amelodentinal and cementodentinal junctions, and formation of pathologic dentin, more frequently in the root than in the crown containing vascular inclusions, abnormal dentinal tubules, and many denticles.

Type III (Familial Hypermobility)

Type III (familial hypermobility) is an autosomal dominantly inherited disorder characterized by marked joint laxity and soft, but minimally hyperextensible or fragile skin and minimal bruising. In the newborn, joint laxity is often striking, although dislocation is rare. Infants may be slow to walk because of joint laxity. Major complications are recurrent dislocations, which may require surgery for stabilization, and early onset degenerative joint disease. Pregnancy and delivery are usually uncomplicated [145]. Approximately 10% of Ehlers-Danlos syndrome patients have type III. The basic defect is unknown [93,94,99,146].

Formerly, type III was known as the benign hypermobile variety of Ehlers-Danlos syndrome [101,102]. However, there appears to be an increased risk of mitral valve prolapse as an associated complication [116,117]. Type III is most commonly confused with normal variant hypermobility found in approximately 4–7% of the general population [147–149]. Horton et al [150] reported an autosomal dominant joint instability syndrome characterized by dislocation of the hip, patella and elbows. Type VII and Type Viljoen also have marked joint hypermobility.

Type IV (Ecchymotic, Arterial, or Sack-Barabas)

Type IV, also known as the ecchymotic, arterial, or Sack-Barabas variety of Ehlers-Danlos syndrome, has the most ominous prognosis because of the predilection for catastrophic bleeding from major arteries and spontaneous perforation of the gastrointestinal tract. About 50% die before reaching 40 years of age [151]. Joint hypermobility is usually limited to the digits, and skin hyperextensibility may be minimal or absent. The skin is characteristically thin and translucent with an easily observed prominent venous network. Minor trauma leads to extensive ecchymosis, resulting in scarring over bony prominences. Musculoskeletal and orthopedic problems do not occur in type IV. The condition is etiologically heterogeneous. Prevalence estimates range from 1/100,000 to less than 1 in a million [93,94,152]. About 35 patients have been reported [151].

Biochemical heterogeneity has been demonstrated and most likely results from different mutations in the same gene rather than in different genes. Type IV results from gene mutations of type III collagen. Mutations have been found that 1) interfere with secretion of assembled molecules, 2) alter the expression of one allele, or 3) lead to increased intracellular degradation of type III collagen molecules. Various skin changes have been observed, depending on the nature of the mutation. Small collagen fibrils and a mixed population of fibril sizes may be present. In patients with defects in secretion, marked dilatation of the rough endoplasmic reticulum is found in fibroblasts [110,152–156].

Both autosomal dominant [93,151,156–158] and autosomal recessive [154,157–159] forms have been observed. Consanguinity was recorded in a family of two affected sibs reported by Sulh et al [159]. In 1979, Byers et al [160] proposed a preliminary classification of type IV with subtypes A, B, C, and D. Subtype IVA has autosomal dominant inheritance and a life expectancy of 30–50 years [157]. Further heterogeneity is known; Tsipouras et al [161] demonstrated different mutations affecting the stability and secretion of pro I (III) chains of type III procollagen in two separate families, both having autosomal dominant transmission. Subtype IVB has autosomal recessive inheritance [154,157] and a life expectancy of 15–30 years. Subtype IVC is represented by a sporadic case in one family; extreme dilatation of the rough endoplasmic reticulum of dermal fibroblasts was noted [160]. Subtype IVD [161], now thought to have autosomal recessive inheritance [159], is associated with collagen fibrils, which are small in diameter but vary in size. As Byers et al [160] recognized in 1979, the classification is heuristic, and it should be anticipated that further studies will result in significant changes. Hartsfield et al [162] found periodontitis in a family with type IV, raising the question of the validity of type VIII.

Temple et al [156], using anti-human type III collagen antibodies, demonstrated the collagen deficit by immunofluorescence.

General features. The skin is thin, inextensible, and translucent (30%), showing a venous pattern over the trunk, abdomen, and extremities and early aging. Minimal joint hypermobility is evident in 30%, being limited to the small joints of the hands and feet. Bruising is marked, and extensive ecchymoses may follow even minor trauma in 65% [151]. Bony prominences are covered with thin, darkly pigmented scars, which differ from those observed in types I and II. The facies is characterized by large-appearing eyes, a somewhat pinched nose, and thin lips [156]. Often, the skin over the face has a parchment-like appearance. Large varicose veins may be present. Patients are at greatly increased risk for arterial aneurysm or dissection (80%), arteriovenous fistulas (20%), spontaneous rupture of the colon (10%), and rupture of the gravid uterus [151,163]. Recurrent abdominal pain without major findings is common and may result from mural hemorrhage in the small bowel. The location of arterial hemorrhage determines the presenting symptoms in some patients (stroke, abdominal bleeding, limb compartmental syndrome), while bowel rupture is the first complication in others. Removal of the distal two-thirds of the colon, the most common site of rupture, may decrease the likelihood of recurrence. Over 40% die prior to surgery [151]. Surgical attempts at vascular repair have been especially unsuccessful because of the friability of vessel walls and other tissues. Usually following prolonged intraoperative attempts to achieve hemostasis, arteries are simply ligated. Conservative treatment, whenever possible, is recommended. Because of the extreme vascular fragility, angiographic studies should be carried out only in the most dire circumstances since complications occur in about 65% [151]. The dramatic, deceptive, and deadly aspects of type IV have been well discussed in the surgical literature. The extreme importance of proper diagnosis of type IV is especially evident when dealing with an undiagnosed patient. In such instances, rupture of an appendix or Meckel's diverticulum, perforation of a bowel by a foreign body, or pelvic inflammatory disease is suspected during surgery for lower abdominal pain. Hemorrhagic tendencies lead to unnecessary and expensive coagulopathy studies. The friability of tissues, development of hematomas, excessive bleeding encountered during surgery, and partial dehiscence of sutured wounds are perplexing to the surgeon [93,94,164–168].

Lifespan is generally shortened. Death has been reported from 12–60 years, most commonly during the 20s and 30s. Causes of death include exsanguination from major artery rupture, sepsis from bowel rupture, and shock from uterine rupture [93,94,96].

The complications of pregnancy, in addition to vascular rupture and uterine rupture, include tearing of vaginal tissues during delivery [118,157, 163,169,170]. Life-threatening complications may occur in 15–20%. In undiagnosed children, easy bruising with minimal or no trauma has resulted in suspicion of child abuse [171].

Other findings. Other findings have been noted on occasion including infantile polycystic kidneys [172], keratoconus, and periodontal disease [93].

Type V (X-Linked)

In 1968, Beighton [173] first reported this entity in two English families. They were reexamined in 1985 [174]. Skin hyperextensibility was striking, but joint hypermobility, most evident in the fingers, was mild. Cutaneous fragility, bruising, and scarring tended to be moderate. Both spheroid and molluscoid pseudotumors were found. There was generalized musculoskeletal weakness (dorsal kyphosis, hernia, pes planus, genu valgum). Clinical features were similar to those affected with type II.

X-linked recessive inheritance was established [93,94,99,101,102, 111,173–175]. Biochemical studies failed to identify any abnormality in the activity of lysyl oxidase, an enzyme involved in crosslinking of collagen [175], and no other biochemical defect has yet been identified [102]. Lifespan is probably normal, and female carriers are asymptomatic [93]. Intestinal obstruction and brain abscess were noted in two male sibs. All affected members of the English families had red hair [174].

Type VI (Ocular)

Among the various forms of EDS, type VI has been the most confusing for us to evaluate. It appears to be extremely heterogeneous. Pinnell et al [176], in 1972, described a form of EDS characterized by low skin hydroxylysine and lysyl hydroxylase deficiency. In addition to the classic features of EDS type I, there were severe scoliosis and fragility of ocular tissues. However, during the past 15 years, a large number of examples have been reported that did not quite fit the definition. Ihme et al [177] suggested three forms of EDS VI: type A—severe with absent hydroxylysine in skin collagen and low lysyl hydroxylase activity in skin; type B—clinically similar but with normal skin hydroxylysine and low activity of lysyl hydroxylase in skin fibroblasts; and type C—principally ocular form with normal biochemical findings. It may be convincingly argued that these groups represent at least three different diseases and thus should not be grouped. However, in most reported cases of type C, biochemical studies have not been carried out. All types have autosomal recessive inheritance. Intermediate values of lysyl hydroxylase have been found in heterozygotes, and prenatal diagnosis is possible [178].

For heuristic purpose we will attempt to define the subtypes as we presently view them.

Both type A [176,178–182] and type B [183–187] patients exhibit loose jointedness with dislocation, excessively stretchable, soft, velvety, bruisable and fragile skin, severe scoliosis, and rupture of the globes and/or retinal detachment. We cannot classify the case of Kuming and Joffe [188]. It would appear to be EDS type IV, but the patient had keratoconus. One family could be either type A or B [189].

Often there is delay in motor development. Height is originally normal but scoliosis develops during adolescence and is progressive.

Epicanthal folds, blue sclerae, keratoconus, keratoglobus, and angioid streaks are common. Glaucoma [182] manifests in the third decade with retinal detachment in the fourth. The cornea or globes may rupture following minimal trauma. Corneal diameter may be somewhat reduced [187]. Myopia, though common, is mild as is hearing loss. Joint laxity can be found in a large number of conditions: *Marfan syndrome, osteogenesis imperfecta, Larsen syndrome, pseudochondroplasia, cartilage-hair hypoplasia,* etc. The osteoporosis-pseudoglioma syndrome has radiologic changes similar to those in osteogenesis imperfecta as well as mild mental retardation, retinal detachment, and ligamentous laxity [190]. Possibly the child reported by Biering and Iverson [191] actually had a form of cutis laxa.

There are numerous reports of type C but again we may be dealing with heterogeneity. Brittle cornea, blue sclera, keratoglobus, keratocornea, and microcornea have been reported as an autosomal recessive disorder in various combinations with or without joint laxity, fractures, macrocephaly, hearing loss, and mild mental retardation [132,191–203]. Red hair has been noted in a few kindred [200,202]. Robertson [204] discovered that 50% of his patients with keratoconus had joint hypermobility. Retinal detachment may rarely be seen in EDS type I [136].

Type VII (Arthrochalasis Multiplex Congenita)

In 1973, Lichtenstein et al [205] identified a distinct type of EDS in three isolated patients. They represented with severe hypermobility of joints with multiple dislocations, especially of the hips, and scoliosis, which in large part accounted for the short stature. The skin was soft, but only mild hyperelasticity and fragility of the skin were observed. The facies was characterized by epicanthal folds, depressed nasal bridge, and micrognathia. Similarly affected isolated examples had been described earlier by Hass and Hass [206]. Several affected sibs in a large consanguineous kindred have also been documented [207]. This recessive form is due to a defective peptidase, which cleaves the aminopropeptide.

The defect in the autosomal dominant form, originally supposed to be due to deficiency of procollagen N-protease, one of two enzymes necessary for the conversion of procollagen to collagen, has been reevaluated [208]. Reexamination of patients with the dominant form has shown various structural mutations of the pro 2 chain of type I collagen that prevent normal enzymatic conversion of the aminopropeptide from the chain [209–212]. Hood et al [213] demonstrated markedly variable clinical expression in individuals with the same structural mutation.

Type VIII (Periodontal)

In 1972, McKusick [94] first identified an autosomal dominant form of EDS characterized by periodontal disease, scarring of pretibial skin unaccompanied by joint hypermobility or hyperextensibility of skin. Stewart et al [214] and Hollister et al [215] reported additional kindreds. In one family, marfanoid habitus, unusual facies, severe skin fragility and bruisability and evidence of visceral involvement (duodenal rupture) were noted. In the other family, normal body habitus and skin fragility but moderate-to-marked skin stretchability were evident. The family reported by Nelson and King [216] had normal facies and body habitus with only slight joint hypermobility. Other examples are less certain [217,218]. Hartsfield and Pinnel [162] have questioned the existence of this type, since they found periodontitis in type IV. We, too, agree that type VIII cases probably represent type IV.

The onset of skin fragility is noted in childhood. Ecchymoses following slight trauma resolve except for the pretibial areas. These heal with tender yellow-brown atrophic wrinkled scars, which somewhat resemble necrobiosis lipoidica diabeticorum or venous stasis. Scarring becomes worse with age.

The periodontal disease appears after puberty, and the permanent teeth are usually lost by the third decade.

Type IX (Cutis Laxa, Bladder Diverticula, Occipital Horns)

EDS type IX, first reported by Lazoff et al [219] in 1975, is characterized by occipital exostoses, soft easily bruisable skin, hyperextensible joints, and widening and bowing of multiple long bones. A number of kindreds have been reported [220–227]. The disorder is due to a defect in copper metabolism leading to lysyl oxidase deficiency and abnormal collagen [220,222–225]. Serum ceruloplasmin and copper levels are low. High levels of copper are found in cultured fibroblasts with low levels in hair. The disorder may be allelic with Menkes syndrome [223,225]. Inheritance is X-linked. It is now classified as a form of cutis laxa.

The face, neck, and trunk are long and thin [220,222]. The hyperelastic, soft, and bruisable skin with resultant atrophic scars and the hyperelastic joints are not as marked as in EDS type I nor as mild as EDS type II. Varicose veins have been noted in 70% [227,228].

Patients exhibit limited extension of the narrow shoulders, elbows, and knees, hypermobility of finger joints, pes planus, and genua valga. Pectus excavatum or carinatum has been found in 40%, and saber skins have been seen in 30%. Various hernias (hiatal, femoral, inguinal) have been noted in about 35%. Bladder diverticula with bladder neck obstruction were found in 60–70%. Chronic diarrhea has been noted in 40% [219,220,222,224,227]. Borderline I.Q. has been documented in 40%.

Radiologic findings include occipital exotoses (horns) symmetrically located on each side of the foramen magnum. These may be palpated, are a constant feature, and may become larger with age. The horns may represent ectopic bone formation within the trapezius and sternocleidomastoid aponeuroses. The clavicles are short with a widened medullary cavity and hammer-shaped distal extremities. The femora exhibit focal hyperostosis at sites of tendon and ligament insertion. Carpal fusion involving capitate-hamate and trapezium-trapezoid coalescence has been noted in over 50% [227,228].

Less specific are deformation of humerus, radius, ulna, tibia, fibula (90%), osteoporosis (70%), narrowing of rib cage (65%), dislocation of radial head (40%), mild platyspondyly, coxa valga, and flattening of acetabular roofs.

Type X (Fibronectin Defect)

Arneson et al [229] in 1980 described four sibs affected with joint hyperextensibility, easy bruising, thin hyperextensible skin, "fish-mouth scarring," but with normal texture. A platelet aggregation deficit resulted in petechiae. While there was resemblance to EDS types II and III, the characteristic velvety skin was absent and striae distensae were common. Petechiae were noted with mild upper respiratory tract infections and often with towelling. The authors suggested that the common link to joint hypermobility and platelet malfunction might be defective fibronectin. However, bleeding was not excessive, and menses were normal. A narrow pelvis [230] and mitral valve prolapse [229,230] have been noted. It should be pointed out that platelet size and function have been demonstrated to be defective in various types of Ehlers-Danlos syndrome [231–233].

Ehlers-Danlos Syndrome, Type Hernández

Hernández et al [234–236] described another variant of EDS. In addition to joint and skin hyperextensibility, increased bruisability, hernia, and papyraceous scars, the propositi had mental retardation, wrinkled facies, short stature, fine curly hair, scant eyebrows and lashes, telecanthus, prominent pinnae, periodontitis, winged scapulae, cryptorchidism, multiple nevi, and varicose veins.

All were isolated cases, but advanced paternal age suggested autosomal dominant inheritance [235].

Ehlers-Danlos Syndrome, Type Friedman-Harrod

Friedman and Harrod [237] reported a mother and son with severe scoliosis, severe hernia, mild joint hypermobility, periodontitis, aortic rupture, and allergic abnormalities (eczema, asthma).

Ehlers-Danlos Syndrome, Type Beasley

In 1979, Beasley and Cohen [238] reported two affected sibs with consanguineous parents. There was hyperelasticity of the skin of the hands, very mild scarring, generalized hyperextensibility of the joints with dislocation of hips and decreased muscle mass. The face was narrow with midface deficiency, small eyes, and possible hearing deficit. One of the sibs had inguinal hernia, cataracts, laterally protruding pinnae, and diarrhea. Both were mentally retarded.

Ehlers-Danlos Syndrome, Type Viljoen

Viljoen et al [239] reported a mother and four children with gross generalized joint laxity, multiple joint dislocations and subluxations, moderate skin hyperextensibility, mild connective tissue fragility, and wormian bones in the skull. The severity of the articular complications and the wormian bones differentiate this from type III.

Differential diagnosis. The term "cutis laxa" has been applied by some authors to the Ehlers-Danlos syndrome. In true *cutis laxa,* the skin hangs in loose, inelastic folds, the voice is deep, and often there are emphysema and hernia. Joint hypermobility may occur as an isolated finding or in association with various disorders such as familial generalized articular hypermobility, *Marfan syndrome, osteogenesis imperfecta, Down syndrome, Larsen syndrome,* and a host of other syndromes. Familial joint laxity has been suggested as still a separate type of Ehlers-Danlos type XI [150].

Laboratory aids. The basic defect can be demonstrated in several types as indicated above. Joint mobility may be tested by the Ellis-Bundick method

[134], and skin elasticity can be tested by the "pinch meter" of Olmstead et al [240] and by the method of Grahame and Beighton [125].

REFERENCES

1. De Barsy AM, Moens E, Dierckx L: Dwarfism, oligophrenia, and degeneration of the elastic tissue in skin and cornea. A new syndrome? Helv Paediatr Acta 23:305–313, 1968.
2. Burck U: De Barsy-Syndrom—ein weitere Beobachtung. Klin Padiatr 186:441–444, 1974.
3. Goecke T, Kiekens R, Majewski F, Pothmann R: Cutis laxa, Hornhautstrübung und geistige Retardierung: Das de Barsy Syndrom. In Spranger J, Tolksdorf M (eds): "Klinische Genetik in der Pädiatrie. New York: Thieme 1980, pp 139–143.
4. Hoefnagel D, Pomeroy J, Wurster D, Saxon A: Congenital athetosis, mental deficiency, dwarfism and laxity of skin and ligaments. Helv Paediatr Acta 26:397–402, 1971.
5. Kunze J, Majewski F, Montgomery PH, Hockey A, Karkut I, Riebel TH: De Barsy syndrome—An autosomal recessive progeroid syndrome. Eur J Pediatr 144:348–354, 1985.
6. Pontz BF, Zepp F, Stoss H: Biochemical, morphological and immunological findings in a patient with a cutis laxa-associated inborn disorder (De Barsy syndrome). Eur J Pediatr 145:428–434, 1986.
7. Riebel T: De Barsy-Moens-Dierckx-Syndrom: Beobachtung bei Geschwistern. Mschr Kinderheilk 124:96–98, 1976.
8. Weidemann HR: Über einige progeroide Krankheitsbilder und deren diagnostische Einordnung. Z Kinderheilk 107:91–106, 1969.
9. Bartsocas C: De Barsy syndrome. In Papadatos CJ, Bartsocas CS (eds): "Skeletal Dysplasias." New York: Alan R. Liss, Inc., 1982, pp 157–160.
10. Bamatter F, Franceschetti A, Klein D, Sierro A: Gérodermie ostéodysplastique héréditaire. Un nouveau biotype de la "progeria." Confin Neurol 9:397, 1949.
11. Bamatter F, Franceschetti A, Klein D, Sierro A: Gérodermie ostéodysplastique héréditaire. (Un nouveau biotype de la 'progeria'). Ann Pédiatr (Paris) 174:126,127, 1950.
12. Boreaux G: La gérodermie ostéodysplastique a hérédite liée au sexe nouvelle entité clinique et génétique. J Génét Hum 17:137–178, 1969.
13. Klein D, Bamatter F, Franceschetti A, Boreux G, Brocher JEW, Holenstein P: Une affection liée au sexe: La gérodermie ostéodysplastique héréditaire (20 ans d'observation). Rev Otoneurophthalmol 40:415–421, 1968.
14. Hunter AGW, Martsolf JT, Baker CG, Reed MH: Geroderma osteodysplastica: Report of two affected families. Hum Genet 40:311–324, 1978.
15. Suter H, Tonz O, Scharli A: Geroderma osteodysplastica hereditaria (GOH) in a girl. In Papadatos CJ, Bartsocas CS (eds): "Skeletal Dysplasias." New York: Alan R. Liss, Inc., 1982, pp 327–329.
16. Wiedemann HR: Geroderma osteodysplastica—What would Virchow have thought about it? Hum Genet 43:245, 1978.
17. Lisker R, Hernandez A, Martinez-Lavin M, Muchinick O, Armas C, Reyes P, Robels-Gil J: Gerodermia osteodysplastica hereditaria: Report of three affected brothers and literature review. Am J Med Genet 3:389–395, 1979.
18. Brocher HEW, Klein D, Bamatter F, Franceschetti A, Boreux G: Roentgenologische Befunde bei Geroderma osteodysplastica hereditaria. Fortschr Roentgenstr 109:185–198, 1968.

19. Gazit E, Goodman RM, Bat-Miriam Katznelson M, Roetem Y: The wrinkly skin syndrome: A new heritable disorder of connective tissue. Clin Genet 4:186–192, 1973.
20. Alibert JL: Histoire d'un berger des environs de Gisore (dermatose hypermorphe). Monogr Dermatol 2:719, 1833.
21. Graf NI: Ortliche erbliche Erschlaffung der Haut. Wschr Ges Heilkd (Berlin) 15:225–230, 1836.
22. Mensing H, Kreig T, Meigel W, Braun-Falco O: Cutis laxa: Klassifikation, Klinik und molekulare Defekte. Hautarzt 35:506–511, 1984.
23. Goltz RW, Hult AM, Goldfarb M, Gorlin RJ: Cutis laxa, a manifestation of generalized elastolysis. Arch Dermatol 92:373–387, 1965.
24. Mehregan AH, Lee SC, Nabai H: Cutis laxa (generalized elastolysis): A report of four cases with autopsy findings. J Cutan Pathol 5:116–126, 1978.
25. Mendoza HR: Cutis laxa. Rev Esp Pediatr 24:735–740, 1968.
26. Siegmund L: Über das sogennante Oedema lymphangiectaticum. Zentralbl Allg Pathol 70:243, 1938.
27. Agha A, Sakati NO, Higginbottom MC, Jones KL, Bay C, Nyhan WL: Two forms of cutis laxa presenting in the newborn period. Acta Paediatr Scand 67:775–780, 1978.
28. Duperrat B, Dufourmentel C, Leis S, Lorenceau B: Cutis laxa et anétodermie. Ann Chir Plast Esthet 22:11–16, 1977.
29. Janik JS, Shandling B, Mancer K: Cutis laxa and hollow viscus diverticula. J Pediatr Surg 17:318–320, 1982.
30. Sestak Z: Ehlers-Danlos syndrome and cutis laxa: An account of families in the Oxford area. Ann Hum Genet 25:313–321, 1962.
31. Weir EK, Joffe HF, Blaufuss AH, Beighton P: Cardiovascular abnormalities in cutis laxa. Eur J Cardiol 5:255–261, 1977.
32. Dallaire L, Cantin M, Melancon SB, Perreault G, Potier M: A syndrome of generalized elastic fiber deficiency with leprechaunoid features: A distinct genetic disorder with an autosomal recessive mode of inheritance. Clin Genet 10:1–11, 1976.
33. Hajjar BA, Joyner EN: Congenital cutis laxa with advanced cardiopulmonary disease. J Pediatr 73:116–119, 1968.
34. Schreiber MM, Tilley JC: Cutis laxa. Arch Dermatol 84:266–273, 1961.
35. Wagstaff LA, Firth JC, Levin SE: Vascular abnormalities in congenital generalized elastolysis (cutis laxa). S Afr Med J 44:1125–1127, 1970.
36. Chadfield HW, North JF: Cutis laxa. Trans St Johns Hosp Dermatol Soc 57:181–189, 1971.
37. Christiaens L, Marchand-Alphant A, Fovet A: Emphysème congénital et cutis laxa. Presse Méd 62:1799–1801, 1954.
38. Goltz RW, Hult AM: Generalized elastolysis (cutis laxa) and Ehlers-Danlos syndrome (cutis hyperelastica). South Med J 58:848–854, 1965.
39. Beighton P: The dominant and recessive forms of cutis laxa. J Med Genet 9:216–221, 1972.
40. Wilsch L, Schmid G, Haneke E: Spätmanifeste Dermatochalasis. Dtsch Med Wochenschr 102:1451–1454, 1977.
41. Balboni FA: Cutis laxa and multiple vascular anomalies, including coarctation of the aorta. Bull St Francis Hosp (Roslyn) 19:26–34, 1963.
42. Brown FR, Holbrook KA, Byers PH, Stewart D, Dean J, Pyeritz RE: Cutis laxa. Johns Hopkins Med J 150:148–153, 1982.
43. Hayden JG, Talner NS, Klaus SN: Cutis laxa associated with pulmonary artery stenosis. J Pediatr 72:506–509, 1968.
44. Lewis E: Cutis laxa. Proc R Soc Med 41:864,865, 1948.

45. Reidy JP: Cutis hyperelastica (Ehlers-Danlos) and cutis laxa. Br J Plast Surg 16:84–94, 1963 (Figs. 10, 11).
46. Talbot FB: Metabolism study of a case simulating premature senility. Mschr Kinderheilkd 25:643–646, 1923.
47. Wiener K: Gummihaut (cutis laxa) mit dominanter Vererbung. Arch Dermatol Syph 148:599–601, 1925.
48. Rossbach MJ: Ein merkwürdiger Fall von greisenhafter Veränderung der allgemeinen Körperdecke bei einem achtzehnjährigen Jungling. Dtsch Arch Klin Med 36:197–203, 1884.
49. Dingman RO, Grabb WC, Oneal RM: Cutis laxa congenita—Generalized elastosis. Plast Reconstr Surg 44:431–435, 1969.
50. Debré R, Marie J, Seringe P: "Cutis laxa" avec dystrophies osséuses. Bull Soc Med Hop Paris 53:1038–1039, 1927.
51. Allanson J, Austin W, Hecht F: Congenital cutis laxa with retardation of growth and motor development: A recessive disorder of connective tissue with male lethality. Clin Genet 29:133–136, 1986.
52. Bittel-Dobrzynska N, Siniecki B: Cutis laxa (Ehlers-Danlos syndrome) with congenital dislocation of the hips. Endokrynol Pol 15:469–479, 1964.
53. Fittke H: Über eine ungewöhnliche Form "multipler Erbabartung" (Chalodermie und Dysostose). Z Kinderheilkd 63:510–523, 1942.
54. Fitzsimmons JS, Fitzsimmons EM, Guibert PR, Zaldua V, Dodd KL: Variable clinical presentation of cutis laxa. Clin Genet 28:284–295, 1985.
55. Goldblatt J, et al: Cutis laxa, retarded development and joint hypermobility syndrome. Dysmorphol Clin Genet 1:142–144, 1988.
56. Hinkel GK, Rupprecht E: Zur Einordnung multipler mesenchymaler Fehlbildungen (Eine Beobachtungen von Dysostosis cleidocranialis mit Dermatochalasis). Arch Kinderheilk 175:292–302, 1967.
57. Karrar ZA: Cutis laxa, ligamentous laxity and delayed development. Pediatrics 74: 903,904, 1984.
58. Karrar ZA, Elidrissy ATH, Adam KA: Cutis laxa, intrauterine growth retardation, and bilateral dislocation of the hips: A report of five cases. Prog Clin Biol Res 104:215–221, 1982.
59. Khaldi F, et al: Cutis laxa. Ann Pédiatr (Paris) 34:165–168, 1987 (Case 2).
60. Patton MA, Tolmie J, Ruthnum P, Bamford S, Baraister M, Pembrey M: Congenital cutis laxa with retardation of growth and development. J Med Genet 24:556–561, 1987.
61. Philip AGS: Cutis laxa with intrauterine growth retardation and hip dislocation in a male. J Pediatr 93:150,151, 1978.
62. Reisner SH, Seelenfreund M, Ben-Bassat M: Cutis laxa associated with severe intrauterine growth retardation and congenital dislocation of the hip. Acta Paediatr Scand 60:357–360, 1971.
63. Rogers JG, Danks DM: Cutis laxa with delayed development. Aust Paediatr J 21:283–285, 1985.
64. Sakati NO, Nyhan WL, Shear CS, Akhtar M, Bay C, Jones KL. Schackner L: Syndrome of cutis laxa, ligamentous laxity and delayed development. Pediatrics 72:850–856, 1983.
65. Theopold W, Wildhack R: Dermatochalasis im Rahmen multipler Abartungen. Mschr Kinderheilkd 99:213–218, 1951.
66. Schirren C, et al: Ektodermale Dysplasie mit Hypohidrosis, Hypotrichosis und Hypodontie. Hautarzt 11:70–75, 1960.
67. Bettman AG: Excessively relaxed skin and the pituitary gland. Plast Reconstr Surg 15:489–501, 1955.

68. Jablonska S: Inflammatorische Hautveränderungen die einer erworbenen Cutis laxa vorausgehen. Hautarzt 17:341–346, 1966.
69. Lally JF, Gohel VK, Dalinka MK, Coren GS: The roentgenographic manifestations of cutis laxa (generalized elastolysis). Radiology 113:605,606, 1974.
70. Cho SY, Maquire RF: Multiple myeloma associated with acquired cutis laxa. Cutis 26:209–211, 1980.
71. Scott MA, Kauh YC, Luscombe HA: Acquired cutis laxa associated with multiple myeloma. Arch Dermatol 112:853–855, 1976.
72. Harris RB, Heaphy MR, Perry HO: Generalized elastolysis (cutis laxa). Am J Med 65:815–822, 1978.
73. Marshall J, Heyl T, Weber HW: Post-inflammatory elastolysis and cutis laxa. S Afr Med J 40:1016–1022, 1966.
74. Reed WB, Horowitz RE, Beighton P: Acquired cutis laxa. Arch Dermatol 103:661–669, 1971.
75. Walshe JM: Congenital cutis laxa and maternal D-penicillamine. Lancet 2:144,145, 1979.
76. Braun-Falco O, et al.: Angeborene Dermatochalasis als Leitsymptom eines Symptomenkomplexes. Arch Klin Exp Dermatol 220:166–182, 1964.
77. Gay S, Dee P: Tracheobronchomegaly—The Mounier-Kuhn syndrome. Br J Radiol 57:640–644, 1984.
78. Meretoja J: Genetic aspects of familial amyloidosis with corneal lattice dystrophy and cranial neuropathy. Clin Genet 4:173–185, 1973.
79. Sakati NO, Nyhan WL: Congenital cutis laxa and osteoporosis. Am J Dis Child 137: 452–454, 1983.
80. Linares A, Zarranz JJ, Rodriguez-Alarcon J, Diaz-Perez JL: Reversible cutis laxa due to maternal D-penicillamine treatment. Lancet 2:43, 1979.
81. Solomon L, Abrams G, Dinner M, Berman L: Neonatal abnormalities associated with D-penicillamine treatment during pregnancy. N Engl J Med 296:54,55, 1977.
82. Hashimoto K, Kanzaki T: Cutis laxa: Ultrastructural and biochemical studies. Arch Dermatol 111:861–873, 1975.
83. Marchase P, Holbrook K, Pinnell SR: A familial cutis laxa syndrome with ultrastructural analysis of collagen and elastin. J Invest Dermatol 75:399–403, 1980.
84. Nanko H, Jepsen LV, Zachariae H, Søgaard H: Acquired cutis laxa (generalized elastolysis): Light and electron microscopic studies. Acta Derm Venereol (Stockh) 59:315–324, 1979.
85. Sayers CP, Goitz RW, Mottaz J: Pulmonary elastic tissue in generalized elastolysis (cutis laxa) and Marfan's syndrome: A light and electron microscopic study. J Invest Dermatol 65:451–457, 1975.
86. Grahame R, Beighton P: The physical properties of skin in cutis laxa. Br J Dermatol 84:326–329, 1971.
87. Rautenstrauch T, Snigula F, Krieg T, Gay S, Muller PK: Progeria: A cell culture study and clinical report of familial incidence. Eur J Pediatr 124:101–111, 1977.
88. Wiedemann HR: An unidentified neonatal progeroid syndrome: Follow-up report. Eur J Pediatr 130:65–70, 1979.
89. Ruden C, Thommen L, Fliegel C, Steinmann B, Buhler U: The neonatal pseudo-hydrocephalic progeroid syndrome (Wiedemann-Rautenstrauch). Eur J Pediatr 147:433–438, 1988.
90. Snigula F, Rautenstrauch T: A new neonatal progeroid syndrome. Eur J Pediatr 136:325, 1981.
91. Martin JJ, Ceuterick CM, Leroy JG, Devos EA, Roelens JG: The Wiedemann-Rauten-

strauch or neonatal progeroid syndrome—Neuropathological study of a case. Neuropediatrics 15:43–48, 1984.

92. Devos EA, Leroy JG, Fryns JP, Van den Berghe H: Wiedemann-Rautenstrauch or neonatal progeroid syndrome: Report of a patient with consanguineous parents. Eur J Pediatr 136:245–248, 1981.
93. Beighton P: "The Ehlers-Danlos syndrome." London: William Heinemann Medical Books, 1970.
94. McKusick VA: "Heritable Disorders of Connective Tissue." St. Louis: CV Mosby Co, 4th Edition, 1972.
95. Denko CW: Tschernogobow's syndrome: A translation of the first modern case report of the Ehlers-Danlos syndrome. J Rheumatol 5:347–352, 1978.
96. Ehlers E: Cutis laxa: Neigung zu Hemorrhagien in der Haut, Lockerung mehrerer Artikulationen. Dermatol Z 8:173,174, 1901.
97. Danlos H: Un cas de cutis laxa avec tumeurs par contusion chronique des coudes et des genoux. Bull Soc Fr Dermatol Syphiligr 19:70–72, 1908.
98. Weber FP, Aitken JK: Nature of subcutaneous spherules in some cases of Ehlers-Danlos syndrome. Lancet 1:198,199, 1938.
99. Beighton P, Price A, Lord J, Dickson E: Variants of the Ehlers-Danlos syndrome: Clinical, biochemical, haematological, and chromosomal features of 100 patients. Ann Rheum Dis 28:228–245, 1969.
100. Beighton P, Grahame R, Bird H: "Hypermobility of Joints." New York: Springer Verlag, 1983.
101. Hollister DW: Heritable disorders of connective tissue: Ehlers-Danlos syndrome. Pediatr Clin North Am 25:575–591, 1978.
102. Hollister DW, Byers PH, Holbrook KA: Genetic disorders of collagen metabolism. Adv Hum Genet 12:1–87, 1982.
103. Byers PH, Holbrook KA: Molecular basis of clinical heterogeneity in the Ehlers-Danlos syndrome. Ann NY Acad Sci 460:298–310, 1985.
104. Byers PH, Barsh GS, Holbrook KA: Molecular mechanisms of connective tissue abnormalities in the Ehlers-Danlos syndrome. Coll Relat Res 1:475–489, 1981.
105. Krieg T, Ihme A, Weber L, Kirsch E, Mueller PK: Molecular defects of collagen metabolism in the Ehlers-Danlos syndrome. Int J Dermatol 20:415–425, 1981.
106. Pinnell SR, McKusick VA: Heritable disorders of connective tissue with skin changes. In Fitzpatrick TB (ed): "Dermatology in General Medicine," 3rd Ed. New York: McGraw-Hill, 1987, pp 1775–1990.
107. Sevenich M, Schultz-Ehrenburg U, Orfanos CE: Ehlers-Danlos syndrome: A disease of fibroblasts and collagen fibrils. Arch Dermatol Res 267:237–251, 1980.
108. Shinkai H, Hirabayashi O, Tamaki A, Matsubayashi S, Seno S: Connective tissue metabolism in cultured fibroblasts of a patient with Ehlers-Danlos syndrome type I. Arch Dermatol Res 257:113–122, 1976.
109. Black CM, Gathercole LJ, Bailey AJ, Beighton P: The Ehlers-Danlos syndrome: An analysis of the structure of the collagen fibres of the skin. Br J Dermatol 102:85–96, 1980.
110. Holbrook KA, Byers PH: Ultrastructural characteristics of the skin in a form of Ehlers-Danlos syndrome type IV: Storage in the rough endoplasmic reticulum. Lab Invest 44:336–341, 1981.
111. Kobayashi T, Oguchi M, Asboe-Hansen G: Dermal changes in Ehlers-Danlos syndrome. Clin Genet 25:477–484, 1984.
112. Sulica VI, Cooper PH, Pope FM, Hambrick GW, Gerson BM, McKusick VA: Cutaneous histologic features in Ehlers-Danlos syndrome. Arch Dermatol 115:40–42, 1979.

113. Fleischmajer R, Perlish JS, Timpl R: Collagen fibrillogenesis in human skin. Ann NY Acad Sci 460:246–257, 1985.
114. Prockop DJ, Kivirikko KI: Heritable diseases of collagen. N Engl J Med 311:376–386, 1984.
115. Vogel A, Holbrook KA, Steinmann B, Gitzelmann R, Byers PH: Abnormal collagen fibril structure in the gravis form (type I) of the Ehlers-Danlos syndrome. Lab Invest 40:201–206, 1979.
116. Cabeen WR, Reza MJ, Kovick RB, Stern MS: Mitral valve prolapse and conduction defects in Ehlers-Danlos syndrome. Arch Intern Med 137:1227–1231, 1977.
117. Leier CV, Call TD, Fulkerson PK, Wooley CF: The spectrum of cardiac defects in the Ehlers-Danlos syndrome, types I and III. Ann Intern Med 92:171–178, 1980.
118. Taylor DJ, Wilcox I, Russell JK: Ehlers-Danlos syndrome during pregnancy: A case report and review of the literature. Obstet Gynecol Surv 36:277–281, 1981.
119. Harris ED, Sjoerdsma A: Collagen profile in various clinical conditions. Lancet 2: 707–709, 1966.
120. De Paepe A, Nicholls A, Narcisi P, De Keyser F, Quatacker J, Van Staey M, Matton M, Pope FM: Ehlers-Danlos syndrome type I: A clinical and ultrastructural study of a family with reduced amounts of collagen type III. Br J Dermatol 117:89–97, 1987.
121. Barabas AP: Ehlers-Danlos syndrome associated with prematurity and premature rupture of foetal membranes; possible increase in incidence. Br Med J [Clin Res] 2:682–684, 1966.
122. Smith CV, Phelan JP: Pregnancy and the Ehlers-Danlos syndrome. J Reprod Med 27: 757–760, 1982.
123. Snyder RR, Gilstrap LC, Hauth JC: Ehlers-Danlos syndrome and pregnancy. Obstet Gynecol 61:649–651, 1983.
124. Owen SM, Durst RD: Ehlers-Danlos syndrome simulating child abuse. Arch Dermatol 120:97–101, 1984.
125. Grahame R, Beighton P: Physical properties of the skin in the Ehlers-Danlos syndrome. Ann Rheum Dis 28:246–251, 1969.
126. Goodman RM, Katznelson BMM, Frydman M: Evolution of palmar skin creases in the Ehlers-Danlos syndrome. Clin Genet 3:67–72, 1972.
127. Benjamin B, Weiner H: Syndrome of cutaneous fragility and hyperelasticity and articular hyperlaxity. Am J Dis Child 65:247–257, 1943.
128. Johnson SAM, Falls HF: Ehlers-Danlos syndrome: A clinical and genetic study. Arch Dermatol Syphil 60:82–105, 1949.
129. Beighton P, Thomas ML: The radiology of the Ehlers-Danlos syndrome. Clin Radiol 20:354–361, 1969.
130. Beighton P, Horan F: Orthopaedic aspects of the Ehlers-Danlos syndrome. J Bone Joint Surg [Br] 51:444–453, 1969.
131. Durham DG: Cutis hyperelastica (Ehlers-Danlos syndrome) with blue scleras, microcornea and glaucoma. Arch Ophthalmol 49:220,221, 1953.
132. Beighton P, Murdoch JL, Votteler T: Gastrointestinal complications of the Ehlers-Danlos syndrome. Gut 10:1004–1008, 1969.
133. Beighton P: Serious ophthalmological complications in the Ehlers-Danlos syndrome. Br J Ophthalmol 54:263–268, 1970.
134. Ellis FE, Bundick WR: Cutaneous elasticity and hyperelasticity. Arch Dermatol 74: 22–32, 1956.
135. Green WR, Friedman-Kien A, Banfield WG: Angioid streaks in Ehlers-Danlos syndrome. Arch Ophthalmol 76:197–204, 1966.

136. Pemberton JW, Freeman HM, Schepens CL: Familial retinal detachment and the Ehlers-Danlos syndrome. Arch Ophthalmol 76:817–824, 1966.
137. Barabas GM, Barabas AP: The Ehlers-Danlos syndrome: A report of the oral and haematological findings in nine cases. Br Dent J 123:473–479, 1967.
138. Goodman RM, Allison ML: Chronic temporomandibular joint subluxation in Ehlers-Danlos syndrome. J Oral Surg 27:659–661, 1969.
139. Thexton A: A case of Ehlers-Danlos syndrome present with recurrent dislocation of the temporomandibular joint. Br J Oral Surg 2:190–193, 1965.
140. Barabas GM: The Ehlers-Danlos syndrome: Abnormalities of the enamel, dentine, cementum and the dental pulp: An histological examination of 13 teeth from 6 patients. Br Dent J 126:509–515, 1969.
141. Gosney MBE: Unusual presentation of a case of Ehlers-Danlos syndrome. Br Dent J 163:54–56, 1987.
142. Hoff M: Dental manifestations in Ehlers-Danlos syndrome. Oral Surg Oral Med Oral Pathol 44:864–871, 1977.
143. Pindborg JJ: "Pathology of the Dental Hard Tissues." Philadelphia: WB Saunders, 1970.
144. Selliseth NE: Odontologische Befunde bei einer Patientin mit Ehlers-Danlos Syndrom. Acta Odontol Scand 23:91–101, 1965.
145. Skovgaard N, Pelle J: Pregnancy and delivery in a patient with Ehlers-Danlos syndrome, type III. Ugeskr Leager 148:2230, 1986.
146. Beighton P, Horan F: Dominant inheritance in familial generalized articular hypermobility. J Bone Joint Surg [Br] 52:145–147, 1970.
147. Biro F, Gewanter HL, Baum J: The hypermobility syndrome. Pediatrics 72:701–706, 1983.
148. Jessee EF, Owen DS, Jr, Sagar KB: The benign hypermobile joint syndrome. Arthritis Rheum 23:1053–1056, 1980.
149. Kirk JA, Ansell BM, Bywaters EGL: The hypermobility syndrome. Ann Rheum Dis 26:419–425, 1967.
150. Horton WA, Collins DL, DeSmet AA, Kennedy JA, Schimke RN: Familial joint instability syndrome. Am J Med Genet 6:221–228, 1980.
151. Cikrit DF, Miles JH, Silver D: Spontaneous arterial perforation: The Ehlers-Danlos specter. J Vasc Surg 5:248–255, 1987.
152. Byers PH: Type IV Ehlers-Danlos syndrome. In Akeson W, Bornstein P, Glimcher MJ (eds): "Proceeding of the Workshop on Heritable Disorders of Connective Tissue." St. Louis: Mosby, 1982.
153. Pope FM, Martin GR, Lichtenstein JR, Penttinen R, Gerson G, Rowe DW, McKusick VA: Patients with Ehlers-Danlos syndrome type IV lack type III collagen. Proc Natl Acad Sci USA 72:1314–1316, 1975.
154. Pope FM, Martin GR, McKusick VA: Inheritance of Ehlers-Danlos type IV syndrome. J Med Genet 14:200–204, 1977.
155. Stolle CA, Pyeritz RE, Myers JC, Prockop DJ: Synthesis of an altered type III procollagen in a patient with type IV Ehlers-Danlos syndrome. J Biol Chem 260:1937–1944, 1985.
156. Temple AS, Hinton P, Narcisi P, Pope FM: Detection of type III collagen in skin fibroblasts from patients with Ehlers-Danlos syndrome type IV by immunofluorescence. Br J Dermatol 119:17–26, 1988.
157. Barabas AP: Heterogeneity of the Ehlers-Danlos syndrome: Description of three clinical types and a hypothesis to explain the basic defects. Br Med J [Clin Res] 2:612,613, 1967.

158. Pope FM, Nicholls AC, Jones PM, Wells RS, Lawrence D: EDS IV (Acrogeria): New autosomal dominant and recessive types. J R Soc Med 73:180–186, 1980.
159. Sulh HMB, Steinmann B, Rao VH, Dudin G, Zeid JA, Slim M, Der Kaloustian VM: Ehlers-Danlos syndrome type IV-D: An autosomal recessive disorder. Clin Genet 25: 278–287, 1984.
160. Byers PH, Holbrook KA, McGillivray B, MacLeod PM, Lowry RB: Clinical and ultrastructural heterogeneity of Type IV Ehlers-Danlos syndrome. Hum Genet 47:141–150, 1979.
161. Tsipouras P, Byers PH, Schwartz RC, Chu M-L, Weil D, Pepe G, Cassidy SB, Ramirez F: Ehlers-Danlos syndrome type IV: Cosegregation of the phenotype to a COL3A1 allele of type III procollagen. Hum Genet 74:41–46, 1986.
162. Hartsfield JK, Kouseff BG, Pinnel SR: Periodontitis in Ehlers-Danlos syndrome type IV. Am J Hum Genet 41:A67, 1987.
163. Rudd NL, Holbrook KA, Nimrod C, Byers PH. Pregnancy complications in type IV Ehlers-Danlos syndrome. Lancet 1:50–53, 1983.
164. Burnett HR, Bledsoe JH, Char F, Williams GD: Abdominal aortic aneurysmectomy in a 17-year-old patient with Ehlers-Danlos syndrome: Case report and review of the literature. Surgery 74:617–620, 1973.
165. Imahori S, Bannerman RM, Graf CJ, Brennan JC: Ehlers-Danlos syndrome with multiple arterial lesions. Am J Med 47:967–977, 1969.
166. Lach B, Nair SG, Russell NA, Benoit BG: Spontaneous carotid-cavernous fistula and multiple arterial dissections in type IV Ehlers-Danlos syndrome. J Neurosurg 66:462–467, 1987.
167. Sparkman RS: Ehlers-Danlos syndrome type IV: Dramatic, deceptive and deadly. Am J Surg 147:703,704, 1984.
168. Sykes EM Jr: Colon perforation in Ehlers-Danlos syndrome. Report of two cases and review of the literature. Am J Surg 147:410–413, 1984.
169. Peaceman AM, Cruikshank DP: Ehlers-Danlos syndrome and pregnancy: Association of type IV disease with maternal death. Obstet Gynecol 69:428–431, 1987.
170. Pearl W, Spicer M: Ehlers-Danlos syndrome. South Med J 74:80,81, 1981.
171. Roberts DLL, Pope FM, Nicholls AC, Narcisi P: Ehlers-Danlos syndrome type IV mimicking non-accidental injury in a child. Br J Dermatol 111:341–345, 1984.
172. Mauseth R, Lieberman E, Heuser ET: Infantile polycystic disease of the kidneys and Ehlers-Danlos syndrome in an 11-year-old patient. J Pediatr 90:81–83, 1977.
173. Beighton P: X-linked recessive inheritance in the Ehlers-Danlos syndrome. Br Med J [Clin Res] 3:409–411, 1968.
174. Beighton P, Curtis D: X-linked Ehlers-Danlos syndrome type V: The next generation. Clin Genet 27:472–478, 1985.
175. Siegel RC, Black CM, Baily AJ: Cross-linking of collagen in the X-linked Ehlers-Danlos type V. Biochem Biophys Res Commun 88:281–287, 1979.
176. Pinnell SR, Krane SM, Kenzora JE, Glimachen MJ: A heritable disorder of connective tissue, hydroxylysine-deficient collagen disease. N Engl J Med 286:1013–1020, 1972.
177. Ihme A, Risteli L, Krieg T, Risteli J, Feldmann U, Kruse K, Muller PK: Biochemical characterization of variants of Ehlers-Danlos syndrome type VI. Eur J Clin Invest 13: 357–362, 1983.
178. Dembure PP, Priest JH, Snoddy SC, Elsas LJ: Genotyping and prenatal assessment of collagen lysyl hydroxylase deficiency in a family with Ehlers-Danlos syndrome type VI. Am J Hum Genet 36:783–790, 1984.
179. Elsas LJ, II, Miller RL, Pinnell SR: Inherited human collagen lysyl hydroxylase deficiency: Ascorbic acid response. J Pediatr 92:378–384, 1978.

180. Krane SM, Pinnel SR, Erbe RW: Lysyl-protocollagen hydroxylase deficiency in fibroblasts from siblings with hydroxylysine-deficient collagen. Proc Natl Acad Sci USA 69:2899–2903, 1972.
181. Krieg T, Feldmann U, Kessler W, Muller PK: Biochemical characteristics of Ehlers-Danlos syndrome type VI in a family with one affected infant. Hum Genet 46:41–49, 1979.
182. Sussman M, Lichtenstein JR, Nigra TP, Martin GR, McKusick VA: Hydroxylysine deficient skin collagen in a patient with a form of the Ehlers-Danlos syndrome. J Bone Joint Surg [Am] 56:1228–1234, 1974.
183. Cadle RG, Hall BD, Waziri M: Phenotypic Ehlers-Danlos, type VI with normal lysyl hdyroxylase activity and macrocephaly. Am J Hum Genet 37:A48, 1985.
184. Judisch GF, Waziri M, Krachmer JH: Ocular Ehlers-Danlos syndrome with normal lysyl hydroxylase activity. Arch Ophthalmol 94:1489–1491, 1976.
185. Quinn RS, Krane SM: Abnormal properties of collagen lysyl hydroxylase from skin fibroblasts of siblings with hydroxylysine-deficient collagen. J Clin Invest 57:83–93, 1976.
186. Sigurdson E, Stern HS, Houpt J, El-Sharkawy TY, Huizinga JD: The Ehlers-Danlos syndrome and colonic perforation. Dis Colon Rectum 28:962–966, 1985.
187. Steinmann B, Gitzelmann R, Vogel A, Grant ME, Harwood R, Sear CHJ: Ehlers-Danlos syndrome in two siblings with deficient lysyl hydroxylase activity in cultured skin fibroblasts but only mild hydroxylysine deficit in skin. Helv Paediatr Acta 30:255–274, 1975.
188. Kuming BS, Joffe L: Ehlers-Danlos syndrome associated with keratoconus. S Afr Med J: 52:403–405, 1977.
189. May MA, Beauchamp GR: Collagen maturation defects in Ehlers-Danlos keratopathy. J Pediatr Ophthalmol Strabismus 24:78–81, 1987.
190. Neuhäuser G, Kaveggia EG, Opitz JM: Autosomal recessive syndrome of pseudogliomatous blindness, osteoporosis and mild mental retardation. Clin Genet 9:324–332, 1976.
191. Biering A, Iversen T: Osteogenesis imperfecta associated with Ehlers-Danlos syndrome. Acta Paediatr Scand 44:279–286, 1955.
192. Arkin W: Blue scleras with keratoglobus. Am J Ophthalmol 58:678–682, 1964.
193. Babel J, Houber J: Kératocône et sclérotiques bleues dans une anomalies congénitale du tissu conjonctif. J Genet Hum 17:241–246, 1969.
194. Badtke G: Über einer eigenartigen Fall von Keratokonus und blauen Skleren bei Geschwistern. Klin Monatsbl Augenheilkd 106:585–592, 1941.
195. Behrens-Baumann W, Gebauer H-J, Langenbeck U: Blaue Sklera-Syndrom und Keratoglobus (okulären Typ des Ehlers-Danlos Syndroms). Albrecht v Graefes Arch Klin Ophthalmol 204:235–246, 1977.
196. Bertelsen TI: Dysgenesis mesodermalis corneae et sclerae. Rupture of both corneae in a patient with blue sclerae. Acta Ophthalmol (Copenh) 46:486–491, 1968.
197. Biglan AW, Brown SI, Johnson BL: Keratoglobus and blue sclerae. Am J Ophthalmol 83:225–233, 1979.
198. Greenfield G, Romano A, Stein R, Goodman RM: Blue sclerae and keratoconus: Key features of a distinct heritable disorder of connective tissue. Clin Genet 4:8–16, 1973.
199. Gregoratos N, Bartsocas CS, Papas K: Blue sclerae with keratoglobus and brittle cornea. Br J Ophthalmol 55:424–426, 1971.
200. Hyams SW, Dar H, Neumann: Blue sclerae and keratoglobus. Ocular signs of a systemic connective tissue disorder. Br J Ophthalmol 53:53–58, 1969.
201. Moestrup B: Tenuity of cornea with Ehlers-Danlos syndrome. Acta Ophthalmol (Copenh) 47:704–708, 1969.

202. Stein R, Lazar M, Adam A: Brittle cornea. A familial trait associated with blue sclera. Am J Ophthalmol 66:67–69, 1968.
203. Tucker DP: Blue sclerotics syndrome simulating buphthalmos. Am J Ophthalmol 47: 345–348, 1959.
204. Robertson I: Keratoconus and the Ehlers-Danlos syndrome. A new aspect of keratoconus. Med J Aust 1:571–573, 1975.
205. Lichtenstein JR, Martin GR, Kohn L, Byers PH, McKusick VA: Defect in conversion of procollagen to collagen in a form of Ehlers-Danlos syndrome. Science 182:298–300, 1973.
206. Hass J, Hass R: Arthrochalasis multiplex congenita. J Bone Joint Surg [Am] 40:663–674, 1958.
207. Capatorti L, Antonelli M: Sindrome de Ehlers-Danlos: Quatro casí accertati a due probabili in una famiglia con piu matrimone fra consanguinei. Acta Genet Med Gemellol (Roma) 15:273–295, 1966.
208. Prokop DJ, Kivirikko KI, Tuderman L, Guzman NA: The biosynthesis of collagen and its disorders. N Engl J Med 301:13–23, 77–85, 1979.
209. Cole WG, Evans R, Sillence DO: The clinical features of Ehlers-Danlos type VII due to a deletion of 24 amino acids from the pro $\alpha 1(I)$ chain of type I procollagen. J Med Genet 24:698–701, 1987.
210. Eyre DR, Shapiro FD, Aldridge JF: A heterozygous collagen defect in a variant of the Ehlers-Danlos syndrome type VII. J Biol Chem 260:11322–11329, 1985.
211. Hood OJ, Horton WA, Duvic M: Ehlers-Danlos syndrome VII caused by an apparent structural mutation in the carboxy portion of pro $\alpha 2$ (I). Am J Hum Genet 41:A100, 1987.
212. Steinmann B, Tuderman L, Peltonen L, Martin GR, McKusick VA, Prockop DJ: Evidence for a structural mutation of procollagen type I in a patient with the Ehlers-Danlos syndrome type VII. Eur J Pediatr 130:203, 1979; J Biol Chem 255:8887–8893, 1980.
213. Hood OJ, Horton WA, Duvic M: Clinical and etiologic heterogeneity in autosomal dominant Ehlers-Danlos syndrome, type VII. Proc Greenwood Genet Center 7:170, 1988.
214. Stewart RE, Hollister DW, Rimoin DL: A new variant of Ehlers-Danlos syndrome: An autosomal disorder of fragile skin, abnormal scarring, and generalized periodontitis. Birth Defects 13(3B):85–93, 1977.
215. Hollister DW, et al: Ehlers-Danlos type VIII. Clin Res 28:99A, 1980.
216. Nelson DL, King RA: Ehlers-Danlos type VIII. J Am Acad Dermatol 5:297–303, 1981.
217. Linch DC, Acton CHC: Ehlers-Danlos syndrome presenting with juvenile destructive periodontitis. Br Dent J 147:95,96, 1979.
218. Piette E, Douniau R: Paradontolyse infantile symptomatique d'un syndrome d'Ehlers-Danlos, un cas sporadique? Acta Stomatol Belg 77:217–229, 1980.
219. Lazoff SG, Rybak JJ, Parker BR, Luzzatti L: Skeletal dysplasia, occipital horns, intestinal malabsorption, and obstruction uropathy—a new hereditary syndrome. Birth Defects XI(5):71–74, 1975.
220. Blackston RD, Hirschhorn, K, Elsas LJ: Ehlers-Danlos syndrome (EDS), type IX: Biochemical evidence for X-linkage. Abst 140: Am J Hum Genet 41:A49, 1987.
221. Byers PH, Narayanan AS, Bornstein P, Hall JG: An X-linked form of cutis laxa due to deficiency of lysyl oxidase. In Bergsma D, Schimke RN (eds): "Cytogenetics, Environment, and Malformation Syndromes." New York: Alan R. Liss, Inc., for The National Foundation—March of Dimes. BD:OAS XII (5):293–298, 1976.
222. Byers PH, Siegel RC, Holbrook KA, Narayanan AS, Bornstein P, Hall JG: X-linked cutis laxa: Defective collagen cross link formation due to decreased lysyl oxidase activity. N Engl J Med 303:61–65, 1980.

223. Kaitila I, Peltonen L, Kuivaniemi H, Palotie A, Elo J, Kivirikko KI: A skeletal and connective tissue disorder associated with lysyl oxidase deficiency and abnormal copper metabolism. In Papadatos CJ, Bartsocas CS (eds): "Skeletal Dysplasias." New York: Alan R. Liss, Inc., 1982, pp 307–316.
224. Kuivaniemi H, Peltonen L, Kivirikko KI: Type XIX Ehlers-Danlos syndrome and Menkes syndrome: The decrease in lysyl oxidase activity is associated with a corresponding deficiency in the enzyme protein. Am J Hum Genet 37:798–808, 1985.
225. Kuivaniemi H, Peltonen L, Palotie A, Kaitila I, Kivirikko KI: Abnormal copper metabolism and deficient lysyl oxidase activity in a heritable connective tissue disorder. J Clin Invest 69:730–733, 1982.
226. MacFarlane JD, Hollister DW, Weaver DD, Brandt KD, Luzzatti L, Biegel AA: A new Ehlers-Danlos syndrome with skeletal dysplasia. Am J Hum Genet 32:118A, 1980.
227. Sartoris DJ, Luzzatti L, Weaver D, MacFarlane JD, Hollister DW, Parker BR: Type IX Ehlers-Danlos syndrome. A new variant with pathognomonic radiographic features. Radiology 152:665–670, 1984.
228. Weaver D: Personal communication, 1987.
229. Arneson MA, Hammerschmidt DE, Furcht LT, King RA: A new form of Ehlers-Danlos syndrome: Fibronectin corrects defective platelet function. JAMA 244:144–147, 1980.
230. Hammerschmidt DE, Arneson MA, Larson SL, Van Tassel RA, McKenna JL: Maternal Ehlers-Danlos syndrome type X. JAMA 248:2487,2488, 1982.
231. Estes JW: Platelet size and function in the heritable disorders of connective tissue. Ann Intern Med 68:1237–1249, 1968.
232. Kashiwagi H, Riddle JM, Abraham JP, Frame B: Functional and ultrastructural abnormalities of platelets in Ehlers-Danlos syndrome. Ann Intern Med 63:249–254, 1965.
233. Onel D, Ulutin SB, Ulutin ON: Platelet defect in a case of Ehlers-Danlos syndrome. Acta Haematol (Basel) 50:238–244, 1973.
234. Hernández A, Aguirre-Negrete MG, Ramírez-Soltero S, González-Mendoza A, Martínez y Martínez R, Velázquez-Cabrera A, Cantú JM: A distinct variant of the Ehlers-Danlos syndrome. Clin Genet 16:335–339, 1979.
235. Hernández A, Aquirre-Negrete MG, Liparoli JC, Cantú JM: Third case of a distinct variant of the Ehlers-Danlos syndrome (EDS). Clin Genet 20:222–224, 1981.
236. Hernández A, Aquirre-Negrete MG, Gonzalez-Flores S, Reynoso- Luna MC, Fragoso R, Nazara Z, Tapia-Arizmendi G, Cantú JM: Ehlers-Danlos syndrome features with progeroid facies and mild mental retardation: Further delination of the syndrome. Clin Genet 30:456–461, 1986.
237. Friedman JM, Harrod MJE: An unusual connective tissue disease in mother and son: A "new" type of Ehlers-Danlos syndrome? Clin Genet 21:168–173, 1982.
238. Beasley RP, Cohen MM, Jr.: A new presumably autosomal recessive form of the Ehlers-Danlos syndrome. Clin Genet 16:19–24, 1979.
239. Viljoen D, Goldblatt J, Thompson D, Beighton P: Ehlers-Danlos syndrome: Yet another type? Clin Genet 32:196–201, 1987.
240. Olmstead F, Page IH, Corcoran AC: A device for objective clinical measurement of cutaneous elasticity. Am J Med Sci 222:73–75, 1951.

Craniofacial Aspects of the Marfan Syndrome

Andrew E. Poole, DDS, PhD

Department of Pediatric Dentistry and Craniofacial Disorders Team, University of Connecticut Health Center, Farmington, CT 06032

The Marfan syndrome is a heterogeneous disorder that has undergone considerable redefinition since its description by Marfan in 1896 [1]. The original condition described by Marfan is not now considered to be the disorder commonly associated with his name but, as we shall see later, describes a variant known as contractural arachnodactyly [2]. I am obliged, therefore, to change the title of my presentation and rather than describing the craniofacial characteristics of Marfan's syndrome, the discussion will focus on the tall, thin type of this disorder listed under the general title of "the Marfan syndrome," a term used initially by McKusick in 1972 [3]. Past authors, however, have not necessarily followed this approach, and this has inevitably resulted in considerable variability in the description of the craniofacial findings. The objectives of this paper are to review briefly the variability in the presentation of the general characteristics of the Marfan syndrome and then to discuss the craniofacial aspects of this disorder as it appears in the literature. Finally, I will present some new information on the bony characteristics of the face in the tall, thin type of the Marfan syndrome.

The Marfan syndrome is a generalized disorder of connective tissue that has a reported incidence of at least one per 15,000–20,000 people [4]. It is generally considered to be a biochemical defect of cross-linking in collagen [5] but with involvement of other connective tissues such as elastin or proteoglycan. No specifically consistent pattern of biochemical findings have, however, been suggested to date [6]. Table 1 shows the general characteristics of the Marfan syndrome. The most consistent findings are those involving the musculo-skeletal system, but cardiovascular abnormalities (98%) and ocular findings (70%) are also frequently found [4]. The condition is generally inherited, and in 85% of cases a positive family history is evident. Of the most common ocular defects, dislocation or ectopically placed lenses is seen in 60% of the patients, with the other abnormalities listed seen occasionally. Anterior chamber abnormalities can be secondary to anterior

Birth Defects: Original Article Series, Volume 25, Number 4, pages 73–81

displacement of the lenses, and this can often lead to glaucoma. Structural embryonic defects, such as colobomata, are rare.

Cardiovascular abnormalities most commonly affect the aorta, which becomes enlarged with aortic regurgitation and dissection. Mitral valve abnormalities, however, are also common.

The most common musculo-skeletal finding is arachnodactyly, which is defined as disproportionately long, thin fingers and thumbs (spider fingers). In addition to long digits, long limbs are also evident in many patients with the Marfan syndrome. The upper to lower segment ratio is generally greater than two standard deviations below the population mean (dolichostenomelia) and the stature is greater than the 95th percentile in three-quarters to one-half of the patients [4]. Abnormalities of the chest wall, especially the sternum, are evident in 68% of subjects. Hyperextensible joints, vertebral column abnormalities, and pes planus are also frequent findings [4]. Particularly noteworthy, from the point of view of this paper, is the craniofacial finding of high narrow arched palate, which is subjectively found in over one-half of the subjects. It is noteworthy that no other specific craniofacial findings are listed here, although dolichocephaly, high arched palate, long narrow face, and prognathism are frequently listed in case descriptions [7–11] and are a common part of a description of the "marfanoid habitus." The data in Table 1 emphasizes the clinical variability in this syndrome, in which some of the major abnormalities are not consistently found in all individuals affected with this disorder. This variability may be a reflection of the genetic heterogeneity evident in the Marfan syndrome. Pope et al have described at least four types of the Marfan syndrome based upon clinical presentation and inheritance pattern [6]. The more common "tall" types of the disorder are inherited in an autosomal dominant fashion. Thin and heavy variants are described. The recessive variants included individuals with a marfanoid-like habitus and joint laxity but often without cardiovascular or ocular abnormalities. The final type, contractural arachnodactyly, is believed to be the disorder originally described by Marfan and is a condition associated with significant joint abnormalities, contractures, and scoliosis. The craniofacial appearance of this variant is not typical of that commonly seen in the "classical" Marfan syndrome [12]. Sanger and Wieman describe the face as having a flattened nasal bridge, deep-set eyes with ptosis, and mild hypertelorism [12]. The nose is small and upturned, and microstomia with retrognathia are evident. The ears have a flattened helix with prominent crura and are described as crumpled. The teeth are often widely spaced with a midline maxillary diastema [12]. Dolichocephaly, high arched palate, and crowded dentition are apparently not usually seen in this variant.

No specific gene markers have yet been demonstrated in the Marfan syndrome, but the use of polymorphisms associated with the various collagen

TABLE 1. General Characteristics of the Marfan Syndrome†

Ocular defects		70%
Ectopia lentis	60%	
Myopia	40%	
Anterior chamber abnormalities	Occasional	
Retinal detachment	Occasional	
Colobomata	Rare	
Cardiovascular defects		98%
Aortic enlargement	85%	
Mitral valve prolapse	60%	
Musculo-skeletal defects*		100%
Arachnodactyly	85%	
U/L segment ratio (<2 SD below mean)	77%	
Pectus deformity	68%	
High arched palate	60%	
Height > 95%	58%	
Hyperextensible joints	56%	
Vertebral column abnormality	44%	
Pes planus	44%	
Positive family history**		85%
Variants include		
Autosomal dominant—tall, thin type		
Autosomal dominant—tall, heavy type		
Autosomal recessive		
Contractural arachnodactyly		
No specific gene markers yet identified		

†Described in the literature.
*Pyeritz and McKusick, 1979 [4].
**Pope et al., 1987 [6].

genes seems to offer the best approach to understanding the heterogeneity [13].

This general description emphasizes the variability in the clinical manifestations of the Marfan syndrome and further suggests heterogeneity. Obviously, this heterogeneity could also substantially affect the frequency of various reported craniofacial findings in this syndrome. Table 2 lists those craniofacial features described from the literature that are considered part of the Marfan syndrome. Subjective assessment of dolichocephaly is reported in 65% of the cases. Dolichocephaly is usually defined as having a cephalic index of less than 75.9 [14]. In most case reports this index was not measured. Clearly, eye defects, especially ectopic lenses, and high arched palate are the most commonly reported craniofacial findings. Jaw size discrepancy (retro- or prognathism) and external ear malformations are seen in at least one-third of all subjects with occasional reports of congenital deafness or

TABLE 2. Craniofacial Manifestations of the Marfan Syndrome*

Dolichocephaly	65%
Ectopia lentis	60%
High palatal vault	60%–75%
Long narrow dental arch	60%
Retrognathism	37%
Prognathism	30%
External ear abnormality	25%
Congenital deafness	6%
Cleft palate	2.5%

*Described in the literature.

cleft palate. The softer, ''gestalt'' aspects of craniofacial appearance that are often seen in the Marfan syndrome are also of considerable importance. This is best illustrated by the role facial appearance plays in the diagnosis of this disorder in historical figures. Abraham Lincoln, Sergei Rachmaninoff, and Mary Queen of Scots variously have been diagnosed with the Marfan sydrome, and in all cases the facial appearance was considered an important observation even in the absence of other ocular, cardiovascular, or muscular findings [15–17].

Quantitative craniofacial data in the Marfan syndrome are not commonly reported. Kurek, an orthodontist who worked with Steve Levin, analyzed the maximum palatal height in 80 Marfan subjects, and these data, which are previously unpublished, are shown in Table 3 [18]. The diagnosis of Marfan syndrome was made from careful analysis of records and pedigrees of patients who had all been evaluated at the Johns Hopkins Hospital. No attempt to subclassify the disorder was made. The cases had not received any orthodontic treatment and were divided into children, i.e., less than 18 years of age, or adults, over 18 years. As can been seen from the data, the Marfan subjects had statistically significant ($P < .05$) greater maximum palatal height than age- and sex-matched control subjects, although the standard deviations, especially in the Marfan subjects, were quite large. Table 4 examines similar data from this study for intercanine and intermolar widths in Marfan and control subjects [18]. To avoid the complications associated with growth, I have only used adults here, but, the data for children were very similar. Statistically significant ($P < .05$) differences were again apparent, with the Marfan subjects having much narrower intercanine and intermolar arch widths than the controls. Evaluation of 35 Marfan subjects for Angles classification of malocclusion, showed that approximately one-third of the subjects fell into each of the class I, class II, and class III categories. This suggests that a class III molar relationship, i.e., lower molars placed more anteriorly, may be more common in the Marfan syndrome

TABLE 3. Marfan Syndrome Maximum Palatal Height*

	Marfan	Control
Children	21.29 ± 3.18	17.74 ± 1.76
Adults	22.95 ± 3.14	20.91 ± 2.37

*Comparison of maximum palatal height in Marfan syndrome and control subjects. Kurek and Levin (unpublished) [18].

TABLE 4. Marfan Syndrome Maxillary Arch Width (Adults Only)*

	Marfan	Control
Intercuspid	32.10 ± 3.35	35.65 ± 2.03
Intermolar	34.70 ± 3.45	41.70 ± 2.48

*Comparison of intercanine and intermolar maxillary arch width in Marfan syndrome and control subjects. Kurek and Levin (unpublished) [18].

than in the general population, since only 10% of "normal" subjects have this type of malocclusion. Bias of ascertainment owing to the method of selection of the Marfan subjects cannot, however, be ruled out.

Case analysis and orthodontic analysis of three patients with the "classical" tall, thin type of Marfan syndrome was recently performed at the University of Connecticut Health Center by the author with the help of Dr. Bhavna Shroff, an orthodontic resident. Only the data from one patient will be described in detail here, but this description is typical of the findings in the other two. Generally, the patients had many of the previously described characteristics associated with the Marfan syndrome including the following:

1. Stature in excess of the 95th percentile
2. Upper to lower segment ratio of 0.83, i.e., greater than 2 standard deviations below the Caucasian population mean
3. Pectus carinatum
4. Arachnodactyly
5. Myopia
6. Mitral valve prolapse with mild aortic dilation

The index case was a female Caucasian who presented with dolichocephaly, having a cephalic index of 66.7. She had a mild anterior open bite with open lip posture and large, narrow hooked nose and long philtrum. She had a very steep mandibular plane with a pronounced chin button. Intraorally her palate was long and narrow (34.0 mm at the first permanent molars). The teeth were very crowded and in a class III molar relationship bilaterally with

TABLE 5. Marfan Syndrome Lateral Cephalometric Analysis (Maxilla and Mandible)*

	Z-scores	
	14 years	17 years
Maxillary length (PNS-A)	−0.7	−2.4
Mandibular length (Ar-Pg)	+0.6	+0.9
Ramus height (Go-Ar)	−4.3	−5.1
Body length (Go-Po)	−0.4	−0.3
Gonial angle (Ar-Go-Me)	+5.2	+5.4

*Z score comparison of a cephalometric X-ray measurement of the maxilla and mandible in a Marfan syndrome subject, at 14 and 17 years of age, with an age- and sex-matched control.

a posterior cross bite. The lateral cephalometric analysis for this patient is shown in Tables 5 and 6. Cephalometric analysis consisted of identification of 53 landmark hard and soft tissue points traced from a standard lateral cephalometric X-ray. This X-ray was taken with the patient's head in a holder such that repeated films could be reproducibly obtained on different occasions. The points were digitized into a computer for comparison with age- and sex-matched controls, using the method of Burstone et al. [19]. The values obtained were expressed as Z-scores, which are the difference between the value for the patient and the mean for the controls, divided by the standard deviation. The points presented here are articulare (Ar), pogonion (Po), posterior nasal spine (PNS), point A (A), gonion (Go), menton (Me), Frankfurt horizontal (FH), and nasion (N) and were similar to those used by Schaedel et al [20]. Table 5 shows Z-scores for measurements of the maxilla and mandible. At 14 years of age maxillary (PNS-A) and mandibular length (Ar-Pg) are relatively normal. The height of the ramus (Go-Ar), however, is very small (Z-score = −4.3). This coupled with a normal mandibular body length (Go-Po) leads to a very obtuse gonial angle (Ar-Go-Me). At 17 years of age, when a mature adult bone age was achieved, the measurements were all similar to those at 14 years with the exception of maxillary length. Here the Z-score dropped from a relatively normal value (−0.07) to a very small one (−2.4). Values for facial profile are shown in Table 6. The lower facial height (ANS-Me) was large, in keeping with the overall appearance of dolichocephaly. The mandibular plane angle (MP-FH) was very obtuse (+5.8), probably a reflection of the clinically obvious steep mandibular plane. The antero-posterior position of the maxilla and mandible yielded significantly negative values, indicating that these bones were retroplaced. Class III prognathism was not evident, indicating the result of tooth position, rather than jaw relationship. Again these measurements did not change significantly between 14 and 17 years of age, although accentuation of earlier trends was

TABLE 6. Marfan Syndrome Lateral Cephalometric Analysis (Facial Profile)*

	Z-scores	
	14 years	17 years
Lower facial height (ANS-Me)	+4.4	+4.5
Mandibular plane (MP-FH)	+5.8	+6.6
Maxilla A-P (N-A)	−1.6	−2.6
Mandibular A-P (N-B)	−3.9	−3.7

*Z score comparison of a cephalometric X-ray measurement of the facial profile in a Marfan syndrome subject, at 14 and 17 years of age, with an age- and sex-matched control.

evident. Similar data for craniofacial findings were also seen in the other two subjects analyzed.

DISCUSSION AND CONCLUSIONS

In order to describe the craniofacial aspects of any disorder it is imperative to 1) define the disorder and its variants, and 2) collect sufficient data about the craniofacial complex in that defined disorder to ensure that it statistically represents the true mean and distribution of variability observed. Additionally, if data from the literature are to be used it is essential to be sure that prior authors agree with the current definition of the disorder or equally carefully describe their own interpretation of that disorder.

Clearly the craniofacial data on the Marfan syndrome from the literature do not follow these criteria. Most past papers are case reports, and wide discrepancy exists in their definition of what constitutes the Marfan syndrome. In addition, little or no attempt has been made to quantify the facial features reported, which would have allowed future comparison between reports. Despite these limitations it would appear that the "soft" signs of craniofacial appearance are of importance in recognizing the Marfan syndrome, especially when other characteristics were not evident or available [17]. While the craniofacial data are not quantitatively reliable or consistently collected from a defined subject population, they do tend to support the concept of heterogeneity in the Marfan syndrome. Without a definitive biochemical or genetic definition of this disorder, however, it is unlikely that the craniofacial characteristics will ever be accurately defined or quantified.

The most serious attempt at quantification of the oral findings in the Marfan syndrome were by Kurek and Levin in their unpublished data described herein [18]. Again, considerable heterogeneity was evident, but nevertheless malocclusion, narrow arches, and high palatal vaults were statistically evident. This observation is confirmed by the data obtained from our patients. Prognathism (i.e., protrusive lower jaw) was not evident, and the class III malocclusion seen more frequently in this disorder was probably the result of tooth position rather than abnormal jaw relationship. The craniofacial characteristics most evident in the tall, thin type of Marfan syndrome were short ramal height, obtuse gonial angle, steep mandibular plane, and long lower facial height. The latter was to be expected with dolichocephaly. High palatal vault and long narrow arches were consistently reported in the literature and were confirmed by measurement in both sets of data presented here. If these data, however, are to be useful in diagnosis of the Marfan syndrome or, alternatively, for treatment of discrepancies in the craniofacial complex, more subjects must be studied and longitudinal growth data must be collected. A study of facial growth patterns in this disorder may be of value in further understanding the role of bone growth in the development of the craniofacial complex, as suggested by Grewe et al in 1971 [21]. An analysis of this kind, however, would be of most value when the genes associated with this disorder have been identified. The role of collagen genes in normal and abnormal bone and soft tissue growth within the craniofacial complex, could then be better understood.

REFERENCES

1. Marfan AB: Un cas de deformation congenitale des quartres membres, plus prononcée aux extremités, characterisée par l'allongement des os avec un certain degré d'amincissement. Bull Mem Soc Med Hop Paris 13:220–226, 1896.
2. Beals RK, Hecht F: Congenital contractural arachnodactyly: A heritable disorder of connective tissue. J Bone Joint Surg 53:987–993, 1971.
3. McKusick VA: "Heritable Disorders of Connective Tissue." St. Louis: CV Mosby, 1972, pp 61–223.
4. Pyeritz RE, McKusick VA: The Marfan syndrome: Diagnosis and Management. N Engl J Med 300:772–777, 1979.
5. Boucek RJ, Noble NL, Gunja-Smith Z, Butler WT: The Marfan syndrome: A deficiency of chemically stable collagen crosslinks. N Engl J Med 305:988–991, 1981.
6. Pope FM, Nicholls AC, Lewkonia RM, Halme T, Dorrance DE, Pomerance A: Clinical and genetic heterogeneity of the Marfan syndrome. Curr Probl Dermatol 17:95–110, 1987.
7. Nally FF: The Marfan syndrome: Report of two cases. Oral Surg Oral Med Oral Pathol 22:715–724, 1966.
8. Fitch HB, Secord RT: The Marfan syndrome. Oral Surg Oral Med Oral Pathol 16:373–377, 1963.
9. Baden E, Spirgi M: Oral manifestations of Marfan's syndrome. Oral Surg Oral Med Oral Pathol 19:757–770, 1965.
10. Kamen S: Oral manifestations of Marfan's syndrome in twins. Oral Surg Oral Med Oral Pathol 21:19–26, 1966.
11. Gazit E, Lieberman M: Severe maxillary arch constriction in a patient with Marfan's syndrome: Report of a case. ASDC J Dent Child 48:292, 293, 1981.
12. Sanger RG, Wieman WB: The C.C.A. syndrome (congenital contractural arachnodac-

tyly): A new differential syndrome for Marfan's syndrome and homocystinuria. Oral Surg Oral Med Oral Pathol 40:354–361, 1975.
13. Tsipouras P: Personal communication.
14. Comas J: "Manual of Physical Anthropology." Philadelphia: Charles C Thomas, 1960, p 316.
15. Young DAB: Rachmaninov and Marfan's syndrome. Br Med J [Clin Res] 293:1624–1626, 1986.
16. Buchanan WW: The arthritis of Mary Queen of Scots: Due to Marfan's syndrome? Clin Rheumatol 5:419, 420, 1986.
17. Schwartz H: Abraham Lincoln and the Marfan syndrome. JAMA 187:473–479, 1964.
18. Kurek RM, Levin S: Comparative analysis of the oral manifestations of Marfan's syndrome: Palatal height, maxillary arch width and occlusion. U of Maryland, Orthodontic Clerkship, May, 1985, unpublished.
19. Burstone CJ, James RB, Legan H, Murphy GA, Norton LA: Cephalometrics for orthognathic surgery. J Oral Surg 36:269–277, 1978.
20. Schaedel R, Poole A, Cassidy S: Cephalometric analysis of the Prader-Willi syndrome. IADR Abstract #2358, J Dent Res 67:407, 1988.
21. Grewe J, Jorgenson R, McKusick V: Model system of craniofacial growth: Marfan's syndrome. J Dent Res 50(Suppl 6): 1501, 1502, 1971.

The Prospective Management of Cervicomedullary Compression in Achondroplasia

Ioan T. Thomas, MD, and Jaime L. Frias, MD

Department of Pediatrics, Bowman Gray School of Medicine, Winston-Salem, NC (I.T.T.), and Department of Pediatrics, University of Nebraska Medical Center, Omaha, NE 68105 (J.L.F.)

Recent reports have emphasized an association between sudden infant death and cervicomedullary compression in achondroplasia [1–3]. The existence of significant neurologic problems is not new, but the incidence of severe complications in infancy and the natural history of the relationship between the neural axis and the skeletal abnormalities in childhood remain an enigma [4,5]. As dysmorphologists and pediatricians, we need to plan for the prospective management of infants with achondroplasia, taking advantage of modern noninvasive techniques to identify those patients at special risk.

Achondroplasia, one of the most common chondrodysplasias, has an estimated incidence of 1 in 26,000 liveborn infants [6]. The term achondroplasia was coined by Parrot in 1878 [7], who described the histologic differences between this disease and rickets. Earlier in this century, the term was loosely applied to include a number of short-limbed dwarfing syndromes, including thanatophoric dysplasia, and was therefore associated with a very high mortality in the newborn period and early infancy [8]. Following seminal publications by a number of authors, the condition became better defined and more accurately recognized [9–12]. In the late 70s and early 80s there followed a period of familiarity, when the condition was seen, at least in childhood, as being relatively benign [13].

More recently, a number of reports have documented recurrent episodes of apnea, quadriparesis, and sudden infant death related to cervicomedullary compression [1,2,14–19]. These authors emphasize the sudden and unexpected nature of these catastrophic complications, and at least one comments on the fact that apnea may be the sole manifestation of medullary compression in children with achondroplasia [15].

Unexplained apnea or sudden unexpected death in children with achon-

Birth Defects: Original Article Series, Volume 25, Number 4, pages 83–90

droplasia was reported by Pauli et al [2]. Eleven of 13 children died suddenly and unexpectedly, and 5/11 showed evidence of acute and chronic compression of the medulla and cervical spinal cord. At autopsy, external signs of compression were severe and obvious in four cases but barely discernible in another. In these five cases, histologic examination revealed pyknosis of neural cell bodies, gliosis, and edema at the level of the foramen magnum [2]. The demographic pattern of infant death in achondroplasia has certain superficial similarities to that seen in the sudden infant death syndrome (SIDS), and in 8/11 cases, death was classified as such. However, these sudden deaths were different from those usually seen in SIDS; for example, 4/11 children died during the day while asleep in sitting positions.

In a recent analysis of a cohort of 701 individuals with achondroplasia, ages from infancy to 80 years, standardized ratios in achondroplasia demonstrated an increased mortality at all ages [3]. The excess mortality in those under 4 years of age was characterized by sudden death, with brainstem compression identified as the cause of 50%.

These major neurologic complications and sudden deaths are better understood if one appreciates the developmental abnormalities of the skull that are seen in all children with achondroplasia. These may be classified as primary and secondary [16]. Primary abnormalities are the result of the abnormal enchondral ossification that characterizes this chondrodystrophy. As a consequence of this, the cranial base is short and the foramen magnum markedly narrowed. Secondary changes represent the skeletal adaptation to the progressive expansion of the brain caused by hydrocephalus. As a secondary abnormality, the cranial vault is large, due to anterior rotation of the frontal bone and posterior rotation of the planum occipitalis of the occipital bone. The size of the facial skeleton is normal, although the nasal choanae may be smaller due to the narrowness of the cranial base. We believe that the anomalies of the cranial base are responsible for the neurologic complications, hydrocephalus, and cervicomedullary compression seen in children with achondroplasia.

The literature contains some contention about the association of hydrocephalus and achondroplasia [20–22]. We feel that there now exists irrefutable evidence that hydrocephalus is commonly associated with achondroplasia—although the degree of ventricular dilatation is variable—and that almost all children with achondroplasia have altered CSF dynamics [21–27].

Reduction in the size of the individual bones comprising the cranial base reduces the diameter of the basal foramina and contributes to the pathogenesis of the hydrocephalus seen in achondroplasia by producing intracranial venous hypertension [24,25]. The cerebral venous circulation returns blood via cerebral veins to the sagittal sinus, which then runs to join with the straight sinus at the torcular Herophili. Blood flows into the sigmoid sinuses and leaves the skull via the jugular foramina to drain into the internal jugular veins on each side. Different investigators have demonstrated venous obstruction at the jugular foramen, and have also shown the relationship between ventricular pressures and the pressure within the sagittal sinus [24,26,28–30]. These studies demonstrate venous obstruction with elevated pressure in the sagittal sinus and dilatation of the subarachnoid CSF cisterns.

Our interpretation of these findings is that venous obstruction at the jugular foramen elevates the intracranial venous pressure, decreases absorption of CSF into the sagittal sinus, and thereby produces communicating hydrocephalus. Some children with achondroplasia may develop non-communicating hydrocephalus with more severe ventricular dilatation, possibly on the basis of obstruction of the fourth ventricular foramina or kinking of the aqueduct of Sylvius.

Stokes et al [17] report a series in which 10% of patients with achondroplasia had severe respiratory complications, including sleep apnea, significant hypoxemia, and cor pulmonale. One of these children, who died at the age of three and a half years, showed compression of the distal medulla and proximal spinal cord.

A further publication provides details of ten patients presenting in infancy with respiratory symptoms and quadriparesis related to a small foramen magnum [18]. Six were treated with foramen magnum decompression and demonstrated immediate postoperative improvement in their respiratory difficulty and gradual disappearance of their limb paresis. Most patients had a moderate degree of hydrocephalus, with dilation of cortical sulci and basal cisterns. The cortical veins were dilated and anastomotic channels were well developed. The transverse sinuses and torculares Herophili were dilated and there was narrowing at the jugular foramina with prolonged circulation time. Two showed a complete absence of drainage of CSF from the exit foramina of the fourth ventricle. In eight cases myelography demonstrated that the foramen magnum was encroached upon by a bulbous odontoid process and the thickened posterior edge of the foramen magnum, both of which compressed the medulla. Radioisotope cisternography showed concentration of the isotope in the sagittal region which persisted for 72 hours and suggested considerable delay in CSF absorption into the sagittal sinus.

Chronic medullary and upper cervical compression may be present as a "silent" lesion because it occurs in an area above the segments forming the cervical plexus and below the medulla oblongata. Signs of root compression in the arms may be absent and the cranial nerves may not be involved [31].

The presence of cervicomedullary compression may be evaluated using somatosensory-evoked potential measurement (SEP). Patients with achondroplasia who have medullary compression have shown increased latency and decreased amplitude above the cervical cord [32]. Of 23 patients with achondroplasia, seven symptomatic patients had abnormal SEPs, the level of abnormality correlating well with the patients' symptoms. Seven of 16 asymptomatic patients had abnormal SEPs with a pattern suggesting cervicomedullary localization; of these, two demonstrated foramen magnum stenosis, and a third, a 6-month-old girl, showed no SEP response above the medulla. She proved to have obstructive hydrocephalus, which was treated by surgical decompression of her foramen magnum and CSF shunting. Five months later her SEP responses had returned to normal and her CT findings were improved.

Three recent studies have attempted to explore the relationship between the abnormal anatomy and function in achondroplasia [5,33,34]. In a comprehensive evaluation of the relationship between cord compression and respiratory abnormalities, Reid et al [34] examined 26 children with achondroplasia, ranging from 4 months to 6 years of age. Most (73%) reported respiratory symptoms such as apnea, pneumonia, loud snoring, or dyspnea. Obstructive sleep apnea occurred in 9/26, and central sleep apnea was also demonstrated in two of these, but neither patient had apnea while awake. Seven patients (27%) had previously known neurologic abnormalities, two with quadriparesis. The foramen magnum was small in 25/26, as assessed by reconstructed midline sagittal CT scan, and 11/26 demonstrated spinal cord atrophy. Bony anomalies of the posterior fossa included a forward extension of the squamous portion of the occipital bone, a thickened posterior rim of the foramen magnum, and dysplasia of the odontoid process. SEPs were normal in nine patients thought to have cervicomedullary compression; all nine had respiratory problems and were subjected to neurosurgical decompression. At operation, all had severe cord compression with atrophy. The results of surgery demonstrated marked improvement in five patients, with one fatality 3 weeks postoperatively.

In a similar study of 32 individuals with achondroplasia, 4 months to 43 years of age, Nelson et al [33] found that 9/32 had a history of apnea and 7/32 had abnormal polysomnography (PSG), four with significant oxygen desaturation and/or bradycardia and three with apnea. PSG was also abnormal in two patients with no history of apnea. One of these had recurrent pneumonia, while the other had no respiratory symptoms whatsoever. Six of the seven with abnormal PSG underwent suboccipital craniectomy because of significant brainstem compression, on the basis of clinical examination, CT scan, and SEP studies. Transverse foramen magnum diameters by CT scan were 4 and 5 SDs below the mean in 90% of those with respiratory symptoms and in 62% of those without such symptoms; similar findings were demonstrated in 83% of those patients with abnormal PSG and in 59% of those with normal PSG. The sagittal diameters showed no differences between the groups. An asymptomatic 14-year-old boy with some evidence of central apnea on PSG and whose foramen magnum diameters were large for achondroplasia was found to have a large posteriorly placed odontoid process causing marked brainstem compression. Daytime apnea sufficiently severe to require resuscitation occurred in 4/32, all less than 18 months old. Three of them had abnormal PSG, and the other had prolonged hypoxemia documented by intraarterial blood gas monitoring. All four had significant foramen magnum stenosis documented by CT scan, abnormal neurologic examination, and abnormal SEPs. At surgery, severe brainstem compression was found in all four, especially in one patient whose spinal cord was thin and transparent at the compressed site [33].

In a study employing magnetic resonance imaging (MRI), 4/5 apparently asymptomatic children with achondroplasia demonstrated compression of the neural axis at the level of the foramen magnum or the arch of C1, with kinking of the neural axis by the posterior margin of the foramen magnum in one child. The fifth child showed anterior indentation of the pons by an abnormal clivus [5]. The authors suggest that MRI scans produce excellent demonstrations of the relationship between the neural axis, the posterior fossa, and the upper cervical spine.

These studies provide a convincing demonstration of the presence of cervicomedullary compression and hydrocephalus in children with achondroplasia. They also suggest that there is a need to place these complications in the perspective of the natural history of the disease process and to introduce a denominator to the numerator they provide. There is no doubt that achondroplasia is associated with life-threatening neural axis compression in some children, but most children with achondroplasia do not suffer from disabling neurologic problems. Many may be in a precarious balance because of the double jeopardy of cervicomedullary compression and hydrocephalus, but the magnitude of the problem and the natural history of the relationship between the neural axis and the posterior fossa and upper cervical spine remain to be elucidated [4,5]. It is difficult to predict which children will develop life-threatening complications.

We suggest prospective assessment of all children with achondroplasia using modern noninvasive techniques. Ideally, the results of these evaluations and the outcome of various interventions should be collected and collated as a collaborative effort of several medical centers. Careful analysis of the data would help to better assess both the natural history of achondroplasia and the relative merits of various therapeutic modalities. We propose the following approach:

All newborn infants should receive appropriate diagnostic studies to confirm the diagnosis of achondroplasia, a neurologic examination, appropriate studies to evaluate apnea, and MRI and CT scan evaluation of posterior fossa and upper cervical spine.

All infants and children older than one month should receive appropriate diagnostic studies to confirm the diagnosis of achondroplasia, a physical examination, and an interview specifically designed to elicit respiratory symptoms such as apnea, snoring, recurrent pneumonia, etc. They should also be evaluated by a pediatric neurologist, looking specifically for signs of neural axis compression (hyperreflexia, ankle clonus, extensor plantar responses, etc.). Sleep studies should be performed, using, if available, a multichannel recorder to monitor EKG, EMG, EEG, transcutaneous oximetry, nasal airflow, rib cage movement, and abdominal movement. Somatosensory-evoked potentials and MRI and CT scan evaluation of posterior fossa and upper cervical spine should also be conducted.

Asymptomatic infants with normal evaluations should be regularly followed and further evaluated as necessary. Asymptomatic infants with abnormal evaluations and symptomatic infants and children with or without abnormal evaluations should be carefully assessed by a multidisciplinary team. Careful consideration should be given to surgical and conservative management options.

Such comprehensive evaluations should not be reserved for the assessment of children with neurologic problems or apnea, but should now be the standard of practice for all infants and children with achondroplasia. There is compelling evidence for increased mortality and mobidity in infancy. Therefore, practicing clinical geneticists and pediatricians should collect more extensive data concerning the incidence and natural history of these life-threatening problems and carefully review the results of various therapeutic modalities. Modern noninvasive techniques can provide such information and should be used in the prospective management of achondroplasia.

REFERENCES

1. Bland JD, Emery JL: Unexpected death of children with achondroplasia after the perinatal period. Dev Med Child Neurol 24:489–492, 1982.
2. Pauli RM, Scott CI, Wassman ER Jr, Gilbert EF, Leavitt LA, Hoeve JV, Hall JG, Partington MW, Jones KL, Sommer A, Feldman W, Langer LO, Rimoin DL, Hecht JT, Lebovitz R: Apnea and sudden unexpected death in infants with achondroplasia. J Pediatr 104:342–348, 1984.
3. Hecht JT, Francomano CA, Horton WA, Annegers JF: Mortality in achondroplasia. Am J Hum Genet 41:454–464, 1987.
4. Wassman ER Jr, Rimoin DL: Cervicomedullary compression with achondroplasia [letter]. J Pediatr 113:411, 1988.
5. Thomas IT, Frias JL, Williams JL, Friedman WA: Magnetic resonance imaging in the assessment of medullary compression in achondroplasia. Am J Dis Child 142:989–992, 1988.

6. Oberklaid F, Danks DM, Jensen F, Stace L, Rosshandler S: Achondroplasia and hypochondroplasia. J Med Genet 16:140–146, 1979.
7. Parrot JM: Sur les malformations achondroplasiques et le dieu Ptah. Bull Soc d'Anthropol Paris 1:296, 1878.
8. Potter EL, Coverstone VA: Chondrodystrophy fetalis. Am J Obst Gynecol 56:790–793, 1948.
9. Maroteaux P, Lamy M: Achondroplasia in man and animals. Clin Orthop 33:91–103, 1968.
10. McKusick VA: "Heritable Disorders of Connective Tissue." St. Louis: C.V. Mosby Co., 4th Ed., 1972, pp 740–856.
11. Rimoin DL, McAlister WH, Saldino RM, Hall JG: Histologic appearances of some types of congenital dwarfism. Prog Pediatr Radiol 4:68–92, 1973.
12. Silverman FN: A differential diagnosis of achondroplasia. Radiol Clin North Am 6: 223–237, 1968.
13. Murdoch JL, Walker BA, Hall JG, Abbey H, Smith KK, McKusick VA: Achondroplasia: A genetic and statistical survey. Ann Hum Genet 33:227–244, 1970.
14. Blondeau M, Brunet D, Blanche JM, Debauchez C, Etienne M: Compression de la moelle cervicale dan l'acondroplasie. Sem Hop Paris 60:771–775, 1984.
15. Fremion AS, Garg BP, Kalsbeck J: Apnea as the sole manifestation of cord compression in achondroplasia. J Pediatr 104:398–401, 1984.
16. Marin-Padilla M, Marin-Padilla TM: Developmental abnormalities of the occipital bone in human chondrodystrophies (achondroplasia and thanataphoric dwarfism). BD:OAS, XIII(3D):7–23, 1977.
17. Stokes DC, Phillips JA, Leonard CO, Dorst JP, Kopits SE, Trojak JE, Brown DL: Respiratory complications of achondroplasia. J Pediatr 102:534–541, 1983.
18. Yamada H, Nakamura S, Tajima M, Kageyama N: Neurological manifestations of pediatric achondroplasia. J Neurosurg 54:49–57, 1981.
19. Yang SS, Corbett DP, Brough AJ, Heidelberger KP, Bernstein J: Upper cervical myelopathy in achondroplasia. Am J Clin Pathol 68:68–72, 1977.
20. Cohn S, Weinberg A: Identical hydrocephalic achondroplastic twins: Subsequent delivery of single sibling with same abnormalities. Am J Obstet Gynecol 72:1346–1348, 1956.
21. Dennis JP, Rosenberg HS, Alvord EC Jr: Megalencephaly, internal hydrocephalus and other neurological aspects of achondroplasia. Brain 84:427–445, 1961.
22. Fowler GW, Sukoff M, Hamilton A, Williams JP: Communicating hydrocephalus in children with genetic inborn errors of metabolism. Childs Brain 1:251–254, 1975.
23. Dandy WE: Hydrocephalus in chondrodystrophy. Johns Hopkins Hosp Bull 32:5–10, 1921.
24. Friedman WA, Mickle JP: Hydrocephalus in achondroplasia: A possible mechanism. Neurosurgery 7:150–153, 1980.
25. Mueller SM, Bell W, Cornell S, deS Hamsher K, Dolan K: Achondroplasia and hydrocephalus. A computerized tomographic, roentgenographic, and psychometric study. Neurology 27:430–434, 1977.
26. Norrell H, Wilson C, Howieson J, Megison L, Bertan V: Venous factors in infantile hydrocephalus. J Neurosurg 31:561–569, 1969.
27. Wise BL, Sondheimer F, Kaufman S: Achondroplasia and hydrocephalus. Neuropediatrie 3:106–113, 1971.
28. Kinal ME: Hydrocephalus and the dural venous sinuses. J Neurosurg 19:195–201, 1962.
29. Shulman K, Ransohoff J: Sagittal sinous venous pressure in hydrocephalus. J Neurosurg 23:169–173, 1965.

30. Weed LH, Flexner LB: The relations of the intracranial pressures. Am J Physiol 105: 266–272, 1933.
31. Blom S, Ekbom KA: Early clinical signs of meningiomas of the foramen magnum. A new syndrome. J Neurosurg 19:661–664, 1962.
32. Nelson FW, Goldie WD, Hecht JT, Butler IJ, Scott CI: Short-latency somatosensory evoked potentials in the management of patients with achondroplasia. Neurology 34: 1053–1058, 1984.
33. Nelson FW, Hecht JT, Horton WA, Butler IJ, Goldie WD, Miner M: Neurological basis of respiratory complications in achondroplasia. Ann Neurol 24:89–93, 1988.
34. Reid CS, Pyeritz RE, Kopits SE, Maria BL, Wang H, McPherson RW, Hurko O, Phillips JA III, Rosenbaum AE: Cervicomedullary compression in young patients with achondroplasia: Value of comprehensive neurologic and respiratory evaluation. J Pediatr 110: 522–530, 1987.

Index